Table of contents

PREFACE

In the hustle and bustle of our modern lives, one fundamental aspect often overlooked is our breath. It is the silent force that sustains us, yet its profound impact on our overall well-being is frequently underestimated. As we navigate the complexities of daily existence, our breath remains a constant companion—effortlessly weaving through the fabric of our existence.

In "Breath Matters: Holistic Approaches to Managing and Improving Breathing," we embark on a journey to explore the transformative power of conscious breathing. This book is not a mere guide; it is an invitation to rediscover the innate wisdom of our breath and harness its potential for holistic health.

Drawing from ancient practices and contemporary insights, this book offers a comprehensive exploration of the multifaceted nature of breath. From the physiological intricacies to the profound connections between breath and mind, body, and spirit, each chapter unfolds a new layer of understanding. Whether you are a novice seeking an introduction to mindful breathing or a seasoned practitioner in search of advanced techniques, "Breath Matters" caters to a diverse audience with practical, accessible, and evidence-based approaches.

Throughout these pages, you will encounter stories of individuals who have experienced remarkable transformations through dedicated breathwork. Their journeys serve as a testament to the resilience and adaptability of the human spirit when aligned with the rhythmic dance of breath. As we delve into the science, philosophy, and art of breathing, it becomes evident that breath is not merely an involuntary bodily function; it is a gateway to self-discovery, healing, and profound states of consciousness.

In a world inundated with stress and distractions, this book serves as a beacon, guiding you back to the simplicity and power of breath. It is an empowering resource for those seeking balance, vitality, and a deeper connection to the essence of life itself. May "Breath Matters" be your companion on this transformative journey, inspiring you to embrace the full potential of your breath and, in turn, live a more vibrant and conscious existence.

Introduction:

Breath is the essence of life. Every inhale and exhale sustains us, nourishes us, and connects us to the very essence of our existence. Yet, beyond its fundamental role in keeping us alive, the breath holds profound significance in holistic health and well-being. In this introduction, we will explore the intrinsic connection between breath and holistic health, as well as provide an overview of various breathing techniques that form the foundation of our exploration.

Significance of Breath in Holistic Health:

In holistic health philosophies, the breath is viewed as more than just a physiological process; it is recognized as a bridge between the body, mind, and spirit. Ancient traditions such as yoga, Ayurveda, and Chinese medicine have long revered the breath as a vital force that not only sustains life but also influences our overall state of being.

When we breathe consciously and with awareness, we tap into the innate intelligence of our body and invite a sense of calm, balance, and vitality. The breath becomes a powerful tool for self-regulation, allowing us to navigate the complexities of modern life with greater ease and resilience. Moreover, studies have shown that conscious breathing practices can positively impact various aspects of our health, including stress reduction, immune function, and emotional well-being.

Overview of Breathing Techniques:

Within the realm of holistic health, there exists a rich tapestry of breathing techniques that have been passed down through generations and across cultures. These techniques offer diverse approaches to harnessing the power of the breath for healing and transformation.
Some of the most commonly practiced breathing techniques include:

1. Diaphragmatic Breathing: Also known as belly breathing, this technique involves engaging the diaphragm to fully expand the lungs, promoting deep relaxation and oxygenation of the body.

2. Pranayama: Derived from the Sanskrit words "prana" (life force) and "yama" (control), pranayama encompasses a wide range of breath control practices from the yogic tradition. These practices include alternate nostril breathing (nadi shodhana), breath retention (kumbhaka), and rhythmic breathing techniques designed to balance and purify the subtle energy channels of the body.

3. Box Breathing: Popularized by modern mindfulness practices, box breathing involves inhaling, holding the breath, exhaling, and holding the breath again, each for a predetermined count. This technique promotes mental clarity, focus, and relaxation.

4. Coherent Breathing: Also known as resonant breathing, coherent breathing involves breathing at a steady rhythm of around five to six breaths per minute. This synchronized breathing pattern has been shown to balance the autonomic nervous system and induce a state of calm and coherence.

As we embark on this journey into the realm of holistic breathing practices, let us approach with an open mind and a willingness to explore the profound wisdom that lies within each inhale and exhale. Through conscious engagement with the breath, we have the power to unlock our innate potential for health, vitality, and transformation.

CHAPTER 1: THE PHYSIOLOGY OF BREATHING

Breath is an intricate symphony of physiological processes orchestrated by the body with remarkable precision. In this chapter, we delve into the intricate mechanics of breathing and explore the profound connection between the breath and various body systems.

Understanding the Mechanics of Breathing

Breathing is a marvel of biological engineering, orchestrated by a complex interplay of anatomical structures and physiological processes. At its core, breathing involves the rhythmic expansion and contraction of the thoracic cavity, driven by the coordinated action of muscles and the dynamic properties of the respiratory system.

The process of breathing can be broken down into two main phases: **inhalation and exhalation.**

- **Inhalation:**
- **The diaphragm:** This dome-shaped muscle located beneath the lungs is the primary driver of inhalation. When the diaphragm contracts, it flattens and moves downward, increasing the volume of the thoracic cavity.
- **Intercostal muscles**: Situated between the ribs, the intercostal muscles assist in inhalation by expanding the ribcage. This expansion further enlarges the thoracic cavity, creating negative pressure inside the lungs.
- **Airflow**: As the thoracic cavity expands and pressure within the lungs decreases, air rushes in through the nose or mouth, down the trachea, and into the bronchial tree, ultimately reaching the alveoli—the tiny air sacs where gas exchange occurs.
- **Gas exchange**: In the alveoli, oxygen diffuses from the air into the bloodstream, while carbon dioxide moves from the bloodstream into the alveoli to be exhaled.

- **Exhalation:**
- **Relaxation:** Exhalation is primarily a passive process, driven by the elastic recoil of the lungs and the relaxation of the diaphragm and intercostal muscles.

- **Recoil**: As the diaphragm and intercostal muscles relax, the thoracic cavity decreases in size. This causes the pressure within the lungs to increase, forcing air out of the alveoli and up the airways.

- **Carbon dioxide removal:** Exhaled air carries carbon dioxide—a waste product of cellular metabolism—out of the body, completing the respiratory cycle.

The mechanics of breathing are finely tuned to ensure efficient gas exchange while maintaining the delicate balance of pressure within the thoracic cavity. The respiratory system's ability to adjust ventilation in response to metabolic demands, environmental factors, and physiological states reflects its remarkable adaptability and resilience.

Beyond its fundamental role in gas exchange, breathing also influences other physiological processes, including circulation, nervous system function, and emotional regulation. By gaining a deeper understanding of the mechanics of breathing, we can appreciate the intricate dance of life unfolding within us with each inhale and exhale.

The Connection Between Breath and Body Systems

Breath is not confined to the respiratory system alone; it serves as a vital link between various body systems, influencing overall health and well-being. The interconnectedness of breath with other physiological processes underscores its importance as a central regulator of bodily function.

- **Respiratory System and Circulatory System:**
- **Oxygenation:** The primary function of the respiratory system is to facilitate the exchange of oxygen and carbon dioxide between the lungs and the bloodstream. Oxygenated blood is then pumped by the heart to deliver vital oxygen to tissues and organs throughout the body.
- **Gas Exchange**: In the lungs, oxygen diffuses from the alveoli into the bloodstream, while carbon dioxide moves from the bloodstream into the alveoli to be exhaled. This exchange ensures the continuous supply of oxygen to fuel cellular metabolism and the removal of carbon dioxide, a waste product of cellular respiration.

- **Autonomic Nervous System Regulation:**

- **Sympathetic and Parasympathetic Balance**: The breath plays a crucial role in modulating the balance between the sympathetic ("fight or flight") and parasympathetic ("rest and digest") branches of the autonomic nervous system. Slow, deep breathing activates the parasympathetic nervous system, promoting relaxation, stress reduction, and restoration.

- **Heart Rate and Blood Pressure**: Conscious breathing techniques, such as diaphragmatic breathing and coherent breathing, can help regulate heart rate and blood pressure by influencing autonomic nervous system activity. By promoting parasympathetic dominance, these practices induce a state of calm and balance.

- **Digestive System and Gut Health:**

- **Vagal Tone**: The vagus nerve, a major component of the parasympathetic nervous system, plays a crucial role in regulating gastrointestinal function and promoting gut health. Deep breathing stimulates vagal tone, enhancing digestive processes, reducing inflammation, and improving gut-brain communication.

- **Mind-Body Connection**: The breath serves as a bridge between the mind and body, influencing emotional states and stress levels that can impact digestive function. Mindful breathing practices can help alleviate stress-related gastrointestinal symptoms and promote overall well-being.

- **Immune Function and Inflammation:**

  - **Oxygenation and Immune Response**: Adequate oxygenation is essential for optimal immune function, as immune cells require oxygen to carry out their protective functions. Deep, rhythmic breathing enhances oxygen delivery to tissues and organs, supporting immune surveillance and response.

  - **Stress Reduction and Inflammation**: Chronic stress and inflammation are closely linked, with stress-induced changes in breathing patterns contributing to systemic inflammation. By promoting relaxation and reducing stress, conscious breathing practices help modulate inflammation and support immune balance.

The profound connection between breath and body systems underscores the holistic nature of respiratory wellness. By cultivating awareness of the breath and incorporating mindful breathing practices into daily life, we can optimize the functioning of multiple physiological systems and nurture a state of vibrant health and vitality.

CHAPTER 2: The Impact of Stress on Breathing

In this chapter, we explore the intricate relationship between stress and breathing, shedding light on how stress affects breathing patterns and emotional well-being. Understanding this connection is crucial for cultivating resilience and promoting holistic health in the face of life's challenges.

How Stress Affects Breathing Patterns

Stress, whether acute or chronic, has a profound impact on our physiological responses, including our breathing patterns. When we encounter stressors, whether they're physical, emotional, or environmental, our body's natural response is to activate the sympathetic nervous system, which initiates the "fight or flight" response. This response triggers a cascade of physiological changes, including alterations in breathing patterns.

1. Shallow Breathing: One common effect of stress on breathing patterns is shallow breathing. This is characterized by quick, shallow inhalations that primarily engage the chest muscles rather than the diaphragm. Shallow breathing limits the amount of air exchanged in the lungs and can contribute to feelings of breathlessness and tension.

2. Rapid Breathing: Another typical response to stress is an increase in breathing rate. Rapid breathing, or hyperventilation, occurs when we breathe more frequently than necessary, often in response to heightened arousal or anxiety. This pattern of breathing can lead to a depletion of carbon dioxide in the bloodstream, disrupting the balance of gases and exacerbating feelings of stress and anxiety.

3. Chest Breathing: Stress often prompts individuals to rely on chest breathing rather than diaphragmatic breathing. Chest breathing involves shallow movements of the chest and shoulders, rather than the deeper expansion of the abdomen associated with diaphragmatic breathing. Chest breathing can exacerbate feelings of tension and contribute to a sense of being "stuck" or constricted.

4. Irregular Breathing: In addition to changes in depth and rate, stress can also cause irregularities in breathing patterns. This may manifest as erratic breaths, pauses or hesitations in breathing, or uneven rhythms. Irregular breathing can further heighten feelings of discomfort and anxiety, creating a cycle of physiological arousal and emotional distress.

5. Dysfunctional Breathing Disorders: Chronic stress and persistent maladaptive breathing patterns can contribute to the development of dysfunctional breathing disorders such as hyperventilation syndrome or breathing pattern disorders. These conditions are characterized by persistent alterations in breathing patterns that lead to symptoms such as breathlessness, dizziness, chest tightness, and panic attacks.

Understanding how stress affects breathing patterns is essential for developing strategies to mitigate its negative impact on overall well-being. By cultivating awareness of our breath and practicing techniques to promote relaxation and diaphragmatic breathing, we can counteract the effects of stress, restore balance to our respiratory system, and foster a sense of calm and vitality. Mind-body practices such as yoga, meditation, and breathwork offer valuable tools for harnessing the power of the breath to navigate stress and promote holistic health and well-being.

The Link Between Breath and Emotional Well-being

Breath is not merely a physiological function; it is intimately intertwined with our emotional state and overall well-being. The connection between breath and emotions is profound, serving as a bridge between the body and mind. By understanding and harnessing this link, we can cultivate emotional resilience, promote relaxation, and enhance our overall quality of life.

1. Breath as a Barometer of Emotional State: Our breathing patterns often reflect our emotional state. When we feel stressed, anxious, or fearful, our breath may become shallow, rapid, and irregular. Conversely, when we are calm, content, or at ease, our breath tends to be deep, slow, and steady. By paying attention to the quality of our breath, we can gain valuable insights into our emotional well-being and inner state of being.

2. Regulation of the Autonomic Nervous System: The breath plays a crucial role in regulating the autonomic nervous system, which governs involuntary bodily functions such as heart rate, blood pressure, and digestion. Through conscious breathing practices, we can influence the balance between the sympathetic ("fight or flight") and parasympathetic ("rest and digest") branches of the autonomic nervous system. Deep, diaphragmatic breathing activates the parasympathetic nervous system, eliciting a relaxation response and counteracting the effects of stress and anxiety.

3. Mind-Body Connection: Breath serves as a powerful conduit for the mind-body connection, influencing both our physical and emotional well-being. By bringing awareness to the breath, we can anchor ourselves in the present moment, fostering a sense of mindfulness and presence. This mindful awareness allows us to observe our thoughts and emotions without judgment, cultivating greater self-awareness and emotional resilience.

4. Regulation of Emotional States: Conscious breathing practices offer a potent tool for regulating emotional states and promoting emotional well-being. Techniques such as deep diaphragmatic breathing, coherent breathing, and mindful breath awareness can help calm the mind, reduce stress, and alleviate symptoms of anxiety and depression. By consciously directing our breath, we can create a sense of inner peace, balance, and equanimity, even in the face of life's challenges.

5. Integration of Breath-Centered Practices:

Mind-body practices such as yoga, meditation, and breathwork offer valuable tools for harnessing the power of the breath to enhance emotional well-being. These practices incorporate breath awareness, controlled breathing techniques, and mindful movement to promote relaxation, reduce stress, and cultivate a deeper sense of connection with ourselves and others.

In essence, the link between breath and emotional well-being underscores the profound interconnectedness of mind, body, and spirit. By cultivating a conscious and intentional relationship with our breath, we can tap into a limitless reservoir of inner peace, resilience, and vitality, fostering a state of holistic well-being that radiates from within.

CHAPTER 3: Conscious Breathing

In this chapter, we delve into the practice of conscious breathing, exploring its benefits and providing techniques for developing awareness of the breath. Conscious breathing is a powerful tool for cultivating mindfulness, reducing stress, and enhancing overall well-being.

Benefits of Mindful and Conscious Breathing

Mindful and conscious breathing practices offer a plethora of benefits for overall well-being, encompassing physical, mental, and emotional dimensions. By bringing focused awareness to the breath and cultivating a mindful relationship with each inhalation and exhalation, individuals can tap into the transformative power of the breath to enhance their quality of life. Below are some of the key benefits of mindful and conscious breathing:

- **Stress Reduction:**
  - Mindful breathing activates the parasympathetic nervous system, promoting relaxation and counteracting the physiological effects of stress.

- By slowing down the breath and extending the exhalation, individuals can elicit a calming response that reduces anxiety, tension, and the body's stress response.

- **Enhanced Mental Clarity:**
  - Mindful breathing helps quiet the mind and enhance focus, concentration, and cognitive function.
  - By anchoring attention to the present moment, individuals can cultivate mental clarity, alertness, and mindfulness, leading to improved decision-making and problem-solving skills.

- **Emotional Regulation:**
  - Conscious breathing provides a powerful tool for regulating emotional states and promoting emotional resilience.
  - By observing the breath without judgment, individuals can create space for acceptance, compassion, and equanimity in the face of challenging emotions, fostering emotional balance and well-being.

- **Increased Self-awareness:**
  - Bringing awareness to the breath fosters a deeper connection with oneself and one's inner experience.

- Through mindful breathing, individuals can cultivate greater self-awareness, self-compassion, and self-acceptance, leading to enhanced self-understanding and personal growth.

- **Improved Respiratory Function:**
- Conscious breathing practices, such as diaphragmatic breathing, help optimize respiratory function and promote efficient gas exchange in the lungs.
- By engaging the diaphragm and expanding the lungs fully, individuals can enhance oxygenation of the body and support overall respiratory health, leading to increased energy, vitality, and physical well-being.

- **Relaxation and Sleep Enhancement:**
- Mindful breathing induces a state of relaxation and tranquility, promoting restful sleep and alleviating insomnia and sleep disturbances.
- By practicing conscious breathing techniques before bedtime, individuals can calm the mind, release tension, and prepare the body for deep, rejuvenating sleep, leading to improved sleep quality and overall restorative rest.

- **Improved Physical Health:**

- Mindful breathing has been linked to numerous physical health benefits, including reduced blood pressure, improved cardiovascular function, and enhanced immune function.

- By promoting relaxation, stress reduction, and overall well-being, mindful breathing practices contribute to a healthier lifestyle and reduced risk of chronic diseases and ailments.

In essence, the benefits of mindful and conscious breathing are multifaceted and far-reaching, encompassing physical, mental, and emotional realms of health and well-being. By incorporating these practices into daily life, individuals can harness the transformative power of the breath to cultivate greater vitality, resilience, and inner peace.

Techniques for Developing Awareness of Breath

Developing awareness of the breath is a foundational aspect of mindfulness and conscious living. By cultivating mindfulness of the breath, individuals can access a powerful tool for reducing stress, enhancing focus, and promoting overall well-being. Here are some effective techniques for developing awareness of the breath:

- **Mindful Observation:**

  - Find a comfortable seated position with your spine straight and your shoulders relaxed.
  - Close your eyes or soften your gaze and bring your attention to the sensation of your breath.
  - Observe the natural rhythm of your breath as it flows in and out of your body.
  - Notice the rise and fall of your abdomen or chest with each inhalation and exhalation.
  - Maintain a non-judgmental awareness of the breath, allowing it to be as it is without trying to change it.

- **Diaphragmatic Breathing:**

  - Lie down or sit in a comfortable position with your hands resting on your abdomen.
  - Inhale deeply through your nose, allowing your abdomen to rise as you fill your lungs with air.
  - Exhale slowly and completely through your mouth, feeling your abdomen fall as you release the breath.
  - Focus on the sensation of your breath moving in and out of your body, emphasizing the expansion and contraction of your diaphragm.

- **Counting Breaths:**

- Sit quietly and bring your attention to your breath.
- Inhale deeply through your nose and silently count "one" as you breathe in.
- Exhale slowly through your mouth and count "two" as you breathe out.
- Continue counting each inhalation and exhalation, starting again at "one" whenever you reach "ten."
- If your mind wanders or you lose count, gently bring your attention back to your breath and begin counting again from one.

- **Body Scan:**
- Lie down in a comfortable position and close your eyes.
- Bring your awareness to different parts of your body, starting with your toes and gradually moving upward to your head.
- Notice any areas of tension, discomfort, or sensation as you scan each part of your body.
- With each exhalation, imagine releasing tension and letting go of any stress or tightness you may be holding onto.

- **Walking Meditation:**
- Find a quiet outdoor space or walk indoors in a calm, uninterrupted environment.

- Begin walking at a slow, deliberate pace, paying attention to the sensation of each step.
- Coordinate your breath with your steps, inhaling as you lift one foot and exhaling as you place it back down.
- Notice the movement of your body and the sensations in your feet as you walk mindfully, bringing your attention back to your breath whenever your mind wanders.

By incorporating these techniques into your daily routine, you can develop a deeper awareness of your breath and cultivate mindfulness in every moment of your life. Whether you're sitting in meditation, practicing yoga, or going about your daily activities, the breath serves as a constant anchor for presence, peace, and well-being.

CHAPTER 4: Deep Breathing Techniques

Deep breathing techniques are powerful tools for promoting relaxation, reducing stress, and enhancing overall well-being. In this chapter, we explore three effective deep breathing techniques: Diaphragmatic Breathing, Box Breathing, and 4-7-8 Breathing. Each technique offers unique benefits and can be easily incorporated into daily life to foster a sense of calm and balance.

Diaphragmatic Breathing

Diaphragmatic breathing, also known as belly breathing or abdominal breathing, is a fundamental technique for promoting relaxation, reducing stress, and optimizing respiratory function. Unlike shallow chest breathing, which primarily engages the muscles of the chest and shoulders, diaphragmatic breathing involves the active engagement of the diaphragm—the primary muscle responsible for respiration. By harnessing the power of the diaphragm, individuals can access a deeper, more efficient breath that promotes overall well-being. Here's how diaphragmatic breathing works and how to practice it effectively:

Mechanics of Diaphragmatic Breathing:

- The diaphragm is a dome-shaped muscle located beneath the lungs, separating the chest cavity from the abdominal cavity.

- When you inhale during diaphragmatic breathing, the diaphragm contracts and moves downward, creating space in the chest cavity.

- This downward movement of the diaphragm allows the lungs to expand fully, drawing air deep into the lower regions of the lungs.

- As a result, the abdomen expands outward, rather than the chest rising upward, during inhalation.

- During exhalation, the diaphragm relaxes and moves upward, expelling air from the lungs as the abdomen contracts inward.

Benefits of Diaphragmatic Breathing:

- **Promotes Relaxation:** Diaphragmatic breathing activates the parasympathetic nervous system, eliciting a relaxation response that reduces stress, lowers heart rate, and calms the mind.

- **Improves Respiratory Function:** By engaging the diaphragm fully, diaphragmatic breathing enhances lung capacity, oxygenation of the blood, and overall respiratory efficiency.

- **Reduces Anxiety**: Deep, slow breaths characteristic of diaphragmatic breathing help alleviate symptoms of anxiety, panic attacks, and stress-related disorders by promoting a sense of calm and grounding.

- **Enhances Digestion**: The rhythmic movement of the diaphragm during diaphragmatic breathing massages the internal organs, promoting healthy digestion and alleviating symptoms of gastrointestinal discomfort.

- **Supports Posture**: Diaphragmatic breathing encourages proper alignment of the spine and improves posture by engaging the core muscles and stabilizing the body's center of gravity.

How to Practice Diaphragmatic Breathing:
- Find a comfortable seated position or lie down on your back with your knees bent and your feet flat on the floor.
- Place one hand on your abdomen, just below your ribcage, and the other hand on your chest.
- Close your eyes or soften your gaze and take a few slow, deep breaths, allowing your abdomen to rise and fall with each inhalation and exhalation.
- Focus on breathing deeply into your abdomen, feeling your hand rise as you inhale and fall as you exhale.

- Pay attention to the sensation of your breath moving in and out of your body, and allow yourself to relax fully with each breath cycle.

- Practice diaphragmatic breathing for several minutes each day, gradually increasing the duration as you become more comfortable with the technique.

Incorporating diaphragmatic breathing into your daily routine can have profound effects on your physical, mental, and emotional well-being. By harnessing the power of the diaphragm and cultivating a deeper awareness of your breath, you can access a potent tool for relaxation, stress reduction, and overall vitality.

Box Breathing

Box breathing, also known as square breathing, is a simple yet effective deep breathing technique used to promote relaxation, reduce stress, and enhance mental clarity. This technique involves breathing in a rhythmic pattern, with equal counts for inhalation, retention, exhalation, and retention, creating a "box" shape with each breath cycle. Box breathing is often utilized in various contexts, including mindfulness practices, stress management, and performance optimization. Here's how to practice box breathing and the benefits it offers:

How to Practice Box Breathing:

- Find a comfortable seated position or lie down in a quiet, distraction-free environment.

- Close your eyes and take a few slow, deep breaths to center yourself and relax your body.

- Begin by inhaling deeply through your nose for a count of four, allowing your lungs to fill with air as you expand your abdomen and chest.

- Hold your breath at the top of the inhalation for a count of four, maintaining a sense of fullness in your lungs without straining.

- Exhale slowly and completely through your mouth for a count of four, releasing all the air from your lungs as your abdomen contracts inward.

- Hold your breath at the bottom of the exhalation for a count of four, experiencing a moment of emptiness and stillness before beginning the next breath cycle.

- Repeat the process, continuing to inhale, hold, exhale, and hold for a count of four each, creating a smooth and continuous flow of breath.

Benefits of Box Breathing:

- **Promotes Relaxation**: Box breathing activates the parasympathetic nervous system, triggering the body's relaxation response and reducing physiological markers of stress, such as heart rate and blood pressure.

- **Enhances Focus and Concentration:** By regulating the breath and creating a steady rhythm, box breathing helps clear the mind, improve concentration, and enhance cognitive function, making it an ideal technique for mindfulness meditation and mental performance.

- **Regulates the Autonomic Nervous System:** Box breathing helps balance the autonomic nervous system, which controls involuntary bodily functions, such as heart rate, digestion, and immune response, promoting overall physiological balance and homeostasis.

- **Provides a Sense of Control:** Box breathing offers a sense of control and stability, allowing individuals to manage their stress response and navigate challenging situations with greater ease and resilience.

- **Improves Sleep Quality:** Practicing box breathing before bedtime can help calm the mind, relax the body, and promote restful sleep, making it an effective tool for insomnia relief and improving overall sleep quality.

Incorporating box breathing into your daily routine can have profound effects on your physical, mental, and emotional well-being. Whether you're looking to reduce stress, improve focus, or enhance relaxation, this simple yet powerful technique offers a valuable tool for finding balance and peace in the midst of life's challenges.

4-7-8 Breathing

4-7-8 breathing, also known as the Relaxing Breath Technique, is a simple yet powerful deep breathing exercise developed by Dr. Andrew Weil. This technique is designed to promote relaxation, reduce stress, and induce a sense of calm by regulating the breath in a specific pattern. 4-7-8 breathing is based on the principles of pranayama, an ancient yogic practice that focuses on controlling the breath to influence the body and mind.

Here's how to practice 4-7-8 breathing and the benefits it offers:

How to Practice 4-7-8 Breathing:

- Find a comfortable seated position or lie down in a quiet, relaxed environment.

- Close your eyes and take a few slow, deep breaths to center yourself and prepare for the practice.

- Place the tip of your tongue against the ridge of tissue behind your upper front teeth, just behind the gumline.

- Inhale quietly and deeply through your nose for a count of four, allowing your abdomen to rise as you fill your lungs with air.

- Hold your breath for a count of seven, maintaining a sense of fullness and stillness in your lungs without straining.

- Exhale slowly and completely through your mouth for a count of eight, making a whooshing sound as you release the breath and empty your lungs.

- Repeat the process, continuing to inhale, hold, and exhale for a count of four, seven, and eight, respectively, creating a smooth and continuous flow of breath.

Benefits of 4-7-8 Breathing:

- **Promotes Relaxation**: 4-7-8 breathing activates the parasympathetic nervous system, triggering the body's relaxation response and reducing stress and anxiety.

- **Reduces Anxiety and Tension:** By slowing down the breath and creating a long exhale, 4-7-8 breathing helps alleviate symptoms of anxiety, panic attacks, and stress-related disorders, promoting a sense of calm and tranquility.

- **Regulates the Autonomic Nervous System:** 4-7-8 breathing helps balance the autonomic nervous system, promoting overall physiological balance and homeostasis by regulating heart rate, blood pressure, and other vital functions.

- **Improves Sleep Quality:** Practicing 4-7-8 breathing before bedtime can help calm the mind, relax the body, and promote restful sleep, making it an effective tool for insomnia relief and improving overall sleep quality.

- **Enhances Focus and Concentration:** By regulating the breath and creating a steady rhythm, 4-7-8 breathing helps clear the mind, improve concentration, and enhance cognitive function, making it an ideal technique for mindfulness meditation and mental performance.

Incorporating 4-7-8 breathing into your daily routine can have profound effects on your physical, mental, and emotional well-being. Whether you're looking to reduce stress, improve sleep, or enhance relaxation, this simple yet effective technique offers a valuable tool for finding peace and balance in the midst of life's challenges.

CHAPTER 5: Breath and Relaxation

In this chapter, we explore the powerful connection between breath and relaxation, highlighting two effective techniques for promoting relaxation: Guided Breathing for Relaxation and Progressive Muscle Relaxation with Breath. These practices offer valuable tools for reducing stress, calming the mind, and cultivating a sense of inner peace and tranquility.

Guided Breathing for Relaxation

Guided breathing for relaxation is a technique that involves using verbal guidance, imagery, and focused breathing to induce a state of deep relaxation and calmness. It is a powerful tool for reducing stress, promoting mindfulness, and fostering a sense of inner peace. Guided breathing sessions are often led by trained facilitators, therapists, or through recorded audio tracks.

Here's how to practice guided breathing for relaxation and the benefits it offers:

1. Preparation: Find a quiet and comfortable space where you can sit or lie down without distractions. Close your eyes and take a few moments to settle into a comfortable position. Allow yourself to release any tension in your body and focus on the present moment.

2. Breathing Awareness: Begin by bringing awareness to your breath. Notice the natural rhythm of your breathing, the sensation of air flowing in and out of your nostrils, and the gentle rise and fall of your chest or abdomen with each breath.

3. Guided Imagery: The facilitator or recording will guide you through a series of soothing verbal cues and imagery. They may invite you to visualize a peaceful and tranquil scene, such as a serene beach, a lush forest, or a tranquil garden. Allow yourself to immerse in the imagery, experiencing the sights, sounds, and sensations of this imaginary environment.

4. Breath Coordination: As you continue to focus on the guided imagery, synchronize your breath with the instructions. Inhale deeply and slowly through your nose, filling your lungs with air. Exhale slowly and completely through your mouth, releasing any tension or stress with each breath.

5. Progressive Relaxation: The guided session may include progressive relaxation techniques, where you systematically tense and then release different muscle groups throughout your body. Coordinate the muscle tension with your inhalations and the relaxation with your exhalations, allowing yourself to sink deeper into a state of relaxation with each breath.

6. Mindful Presence: Throughout the guided session, maintain a sense of mindful presence and awareness of your breath. Notice any thoughts, sensations, or emotions that arise without judgment, allowing them to come and go like passing clouds in the sky.

7. Closing: As the guided session comes to an end, gradually transition back to your everyday awareness. Take a few moments to savor the feelings of relaxation and calmness that arise. When you are ready, gently open your eyes and return to the present moment, feeling refreshed and rejuvenated.

Benefits of Guided Breathing for Relaxation:
- Promotes deep relaxation and stress reduction
- Cultivates mindfulness and present moment awareness
- Enhances self-awareness and emotional regulation
- Facilitates a sense of inner peace and well-being
- Improves sleep quality and aids in insomnia relief

Guided breathing for relaxation offers a simple yet powerful way to unwind, recharge, and find balance amidst the demands of daily life. Whether practiced independently or with the guidance of a facilitator or recording, it provides a valuable tool for managing stress, promoting relaxation, and enhancing overall well-being.

Progressive Muscle Relaxation with Breath

Progressive Muscle Relaxation (PMR) with Breath is a relaxation technique that combines deep breathing with the systematic tensing and releasing of different muscle groups throughout the body. This method is highly effective in reducing physical tension, alleviating stress, and promoting overall relaxation. By pairing breath awareness with muscle relaxation, individuals can enhance their mind-body connection and achieve a profound state of calmness.

Here's how to practice Progressive Muscle Relaxation with Breath and the benefits it offers:

1. Preparation: Find a quiet and comfortable space where you can sit or lie down without interruptions. Close your eyes and take a few moments to center yourself and bring awareness to your breath. Allow yourself to release any tension in your body and prepare for the practice.

2. Breath Coordination: Begin by focusing on your breath. Inhale deeply and slowly through your nose, allowing your abdomen to rise as you fill your lungs with air. Exhale slowly and completely through your mouth, releasing any tension or stress with each breath. Continue to breathe deeply and rhythmically throughout the practice.

3. Muscle Tension: Starting with your toes, tense the muscles in one area of your body while inhaling deeply. Hold the tension for a few seconds, allowing yourself to feel the sensations of tightness and contraction. As you exhale slowly and completely, release the tension in the muscles, allowing them to relax fully and sink into a state of softness and ease.

4. Progressive Relaxation: Move systematically through different muscle groups in your body, tensing and then releasing each area as you coordinate your breath. Progress from your feet to your calves, thighs, buttocks, abdomen, chest, arms, shoulders, neck, and face. Focus on each muscle group individually, allowing yourself to fully experience the contrast between tension and relaxation.

5. Mindful Awareness: Throughout the practice, maintain a sense of mindful awareness and presence. Notice any sensations, thoughts, or emotions that arise without judgment, allowing them to come and go like passing clouds in the sky. Stay connected to your breath and the sensations in your body, using each exhalation as an opportunity to release tension and let go.

6. Closing: As you complete the progressive muscle relaxation sequence, take a few moments to rest and savor the feelings of relaxation and calmness that arise. Notice how your body feels lighter, more relaxed, and at ease. When you are ready, gently open your eyes and return to the present moment, feeling refreshed and rejuvenated.

Benefits of Progressive Muscle Relaxation with Breath:
- Relieves physical tension and muscle stiffness
- Promotes deep relaxation and stress relief
- Enhances body awareness and mindfulness
- Facilitates improved posture and flexibility
- Reduces symptoms of anxiety, insomnia, and chronic pain

Progressive Muscle Relaxation with Breath offers a simple yet effective way to unwind, release tension, and restore balance to the body and mind. Whether practiced independently or guided by a facilitator, it provides a valuable tool for managing stress, promoting relaxation, and enhancing overall well-being.

CHAPTER 6: Yogic Breathing Practices (Pranayama)

In this chapter, we delve into the ancient art of Pranayama, which is the practice of breath control in yoga. Pranayama techniques offer profound benefits for physical health, mental clarity, and spiritual growth. We explore the fundamentals of Pranayama and specific techniques for various purposes, empowering individuals to harness the power of breath to enhance their well-being.

Introduction to Pranayama

Pranayama, an integral aspect of yoga, is the ancient practice of breath control. The term "Pranayama" is derived from two Sanskrit words: "prana," meaning life force or vital energy, and "ayama," meaning expansion or extension. Together, Pranayama signifies the expansion and regulation of the life force through the breath. It is a fundamental aspect of yoga philosophy and is believed to be a pathway to inner peace, self-awareness, and spiritual awakening.

In yogic tradition, the breath is regarded as a bridge between the body and the mind, linking the physical and subtle energies of the human system. Prana, often likened to the concept of qi or chi in other Eastern traditions, is considered the vital energy that animates all living beings. By consciously controlling the breath, practitioners can influence the flow of prana within the body, promoting health, balance, and harmony on all levels—physical, mental, emotional, and spiritual.

The practice of Pranayama encompasses a wide range of techniques, each with its own unique effects and purposes. Some Pranayama practices focus on regulating the rhythm, depth, and duration of the breath, while others involve specific patterns of inhalation, exhalation, and retention. Through regular practice, practitioners can refine their breath control skills, increase their lung capacity, and cultivate a deeper connection to the life force within and around them.

Benefits of Pranayama practice include:

1. Physical Health: Pranayama techniques help improve respiratory function, increase oxygenation of the blood, and enhance overall lung capacity. Regular practice can alleviate respiratory disorders, strengthen the immune system, and promote vitality and longevity.

2. Mental Clarity: By calming the mind and reducing mental chatter, Pranayama practices foster clarity, focus, and concentration. They help quiet the fluctuations of the mind (chitta vritti) and cultivate a state of inner peace and equanimity.

3. Emotional Balance: Pranayama techniques have a profound effect on the nervous system, promoting relaxation and reducing stress and anxiety. They help regulate the autonomic nervous system, balance the sympathetic and parasympathetic branches, and promote emotional stability and resilience.

4. Spiritual Growth: In yogic tradition, Pranayama is considered a powerful tool for spiritual growth and self-realization. By purifying the subtle energy channels (nadis) and awakening the dormant spiritual energy (kundalini), Pranayama practices facilitate spiritual awakening, inner transformation, and union with the divine.

While Pranayama is an ancient practice rooted in yoga philosophy, its relevance and applicability extend far beyond the confines of the yoga mat. In today's fast-paced world, where stress and distractions abound, cultivating a conscious relationship with the breath can be a gateway to health, peace, and inner fulfillment. Whether practiced as part of a comprehensive yoga regimen or integrated into daily life, Pranayama offers a timeless and invaluable tool for holistic well-being and self-discovery.

Specific Pranayama Techniques for Various Purposes

Pranayama, the art of breath control, encompasses a diverse range of techniques that serve various purposes, from promoting physical health to facilitating mental clarity and spiritual growth. Each Pranayama technique has its own unique effects on the body, mind, and spirit, making them versatile tools for enhancing overall well-being.

Here are some specific Pranayama techniques and their respective purposes:

1. Nadi Shodhana (Alternate Nostril Breathing):

- **Purpose:** Nadi Shodhana balances the flow of energy in the subtle energy channels (nadis) and purifies the energy channels in the body.

- **Technique:** Alternate nostril breathing involves inhaling through one nostril while closing the other nostril with the thumb, then exhaling through the opposite nostril while closing the first nostril with the ring finger. This alternating pattern is repeated for several rounds, promoting balance and harmony in the body and mind.

2. Ujjayi Pranayama (Victorious Breath):

- **Purpose:** Ujjayi Pranayama increases internal heat, builds energy, and fosters concentration and mindfulness during yoga practice.

- **Technique:** Ujjayi Pranayama involves constricting the back of the throat slightly to create a soft, ocean-like sound during both inhalation and exhalation. This audible breath helps deepen the breath, regulate its rhythm, and anchor the mind in the present moment.

3. Bhramari Pranayama (Humming Bee Breath):

- **Purpose:** Bhramari Pranayama calms the mind, relieves stress and anxiety, and promotes inner peace and tranquility.

- **Technique:** Bhramari Pranayama is performed by inhaling deeply and then exhaling slowly while making a soft humming sound, similar to the buzzing of a bee. This soothing vibration resonates within the body, calming the nervous system and inducing a state of relaxation.

4. Kapalabhati Pranayama (Skull-Shining Breath):

- **Purpose:** Kapalabhati Pranayama purifies the respiratory system, increases energy levels, and stimulates the digestive fire (agni) in the abdomen.

- **Technique:** Kapalabhati Pranayama involves rapid, forceful exhalations through the nose, followed by passive inhalations. The emphasis is on the exhalation, which is generated by a quick contraction of the abdominal muscles. This dynamic breath cleanses the lungs, invigorates the body, and awakens dormant energy.

5. Sheetali Pranayama (Cooling Breath):

- **Purpose:** Sheetali Pranayama cools the body, calms the mind, and reduces excess heat or Pitta dosha in the system.

- **Technique:** Sheetali Pranayama is performed by curling the sides of the tongue into a tube shape and inhaling deeply through the mouth, then exhaling slowly through the nose. This breath creates a cooling sensation in the body, soothes the nervous system, and balances internal heat.

6. Bhastrika Pranayama (Bellows Breath):

- **Purpose:** Bhastrika Pranayama increases vitality, boosts energy levels, and stimulates the flow of prana throughout the body.

- **Technique:** Bhastrika Pranayama involves rapid, forceful inhalations and exhalations through the nose, with equal emphasis on both the inhalation and exhalation. The breath is quick and powerful, resembling the pumping action of a bellows. This dynamic breath generates heat, purifies the respiratory system, and invigorates the entire being.

7. Anulom Vilom Pranayama (Alternate Nostril Breathing):

- **Purpose:** Anulom Vilom Pranayama balances the flow of prana, calms the mind, and promotes mental clarity and focus.

- **Technique:** Anulom Vilom Pranayama involves alternating the breath between the left and right nostrils using the thumb and ring finger. With the right hand, the practitioner closes one nostril while inhaling through the other, then switches nostrils and exhales through the opposite side. This alternating breath pattern balances the flow of energy in the body and harmonizes the nervous system.

These are just a few examples of the many Pranayama techniques available in the yogic tradition. Each technique offers unique benefits and effects on the body, mind, and spirit, making them valuable tools for enhancing overall well-being and cultivating a deeper connection to the breath and life force within. Whether practiced independently or as part of a yoga regimen, Pranayama techniques provide a pathway to health, vitality, and inner peace.

CHAPTER 7: Breath and Meditation

Breath and meditation are deeply intertwined practices that have been utilized for centuries to cultivate mindfulness, enhance self-awareness, and promote inner peace. In this chapter, we explore the integration of breath into meditation and introduce mindfulness meditation with a focus on the breath.

Incorporating Breath into Meditation

Incorporating breath into meditation is a foundational practice that has been utilized across various contemplative traditions for centuries. The breath serves as a potent anchor for the mind, allowing practitioners to cultivate present-moment awareness, inner peace, and clarity of mind.

Here's an exploration of how to incorporate breath into meditation:

1. Establishing a Comfortable Posture: Begin by finding a comfortable seated position, either on a cushion or chair, with your spine erect and shoulders relaxed. You can also choose to lie down if that's more comfortable for you. The key is to find a posture that allows you to be relaxed yet alert.

2. Bringing Attention to the Breath: Close your eyes gently and bring your awareness to the natural rhythm of your breath. Notice the sensations of the breath as it flows in and out of your body. You may feel the rising and falling of your chest or the expansion and contraction of your abdomen. Simply observe these sensations without trying to control or manipulate the breath in any way.

3. Using the Breath as an Anchor: As you continue to breathe, use the breath as an anchor for your attention. Whenever you notice your mind wandering to thoughts, emotions, or sensations, gently bring your focus back to the breath. You can do this by simply noting "in" as you inhale and "out" as you exhale, or by counting the breaths if that helps maintain your focus.

4. Cultivating Mindfulness: Allow your awareness to rest fully on the breath, moment by moment. Notice the subtleties of each breath—the temperature, the texture, the length of the inhale and exhale. As you cultivate mindfulness of the breath, you may begin to notice the space between thoughts, the stillness within you, and the vastness of your own awareness.

5. Acceptance and Non-Judgment: As you practice, it's natural for your mind to wander. When this happens, simply acknowledge it with kindness and without judgment, and gently guide your attention back to the breath. Remember that the nature of the mind is to wander, and the practice is simply to notice and return, over and over again.

6. Deepening the Practice: As you become more comfortable with incorporating breath into your meditation practice, you can experiment with different techniques, such as deepening the breath, lengthening the exhale, or exploring different areas of the body where you feel the breath most prominently. You can also explore various breath-based meditation techniques from different traditions, such as mindfulness of breathing (Anapanasati) in Buddhist meditation or pranayama in yoga.

7. Integrating Breath with Other Meditation Practices: Finally, you can explore how breath can complement other meditation practices, such as loving-kindness meditation, body scan meditation, or visualization practices. By incorporating breath into these practices, you can deepen your experience and cultivate greater levels of presence and insight.

Incorporating breath into meditation is a simple yet profound practice that can transform your relationship with your mind, body, and spirit. By cultivating mindfulness of the breath, you can develop greater clarity, peace, and resilience in the face of life's challenges, and tap into the innate wisdom and compassion that lies within you.

Mindfulness Meditation with Breath Focus

Mindfulness meditation with a focus on the breath is a foundational practice in many contemplative traditions, including Buddhism and modern mindfulness-based approaches. It involves cultivating present-moment awareness by using the breath as a focal point for attention. This practice helps to quiet the mind, develop concentration, and foster a deep sense of inner calm and clarity.

Here's how to engage in mindfulness meditation with a focus on the breath:

1. Settle into a Comfortable Position: Find a quiet and comfortable place to sit or lie down. You can sit cross-legged on a cushion or chair with your back straight but relaxed. Alternatively, you can lie down on your back with your arms by your sides and legs uncrossed. The key is to find a position that allows you to be both alert and relaxed.

2. Close Your Eyes or Soften Your Gaze: Close your eyes gently to reduce visual distractions, or if you prefer, you can keep them open with a soft gaze directed downward. This helps to direct your attention inward and cultivate a sense of inner awareness.

3. Bring Attention to the Breath: Begin by bringing your attention to the sensation of the breath in your body. Notice the rising and falling of your chest or abdomen with each inhale and exhale. You can also focus on the sensation of the breath as it passes through your nostrils or the gentle expansion and contraction of your belly.

4. Anchor Your Attention: Use the breath as an anchor for your attention. Whenever you notice your mind wandering to thoughts, emotions, or sensations, gently bring your focus back to the breath. You can do this by simply observing the breath without judgment or analysis, allowing each inhale and exhale to unfold naturally.

5. Cultivate Non-Judgmental Awareness: As you continue to focus on the breath, practice cultivating a sense of non-judgmental awareness. Notice any thoughts, feelings, or sensations that arise without getting caught up in them or trying to change them. Simply observe them with curiosity and kindness, allowing them to come and go like passing clouds in the sky.

6. Stay Present in the Moment: Remain present with the breath, moment by moment. You may notice that your mind wanders frequently, which is natural and to be expected. When this happens, gently acknowledge the distraction and return your attention back to the breath, without self-criticism or frustration.

7. Practice Continuously: Continue to practice mindfulness meditation with breath focus for a predetermined period of time, such as 10 to 20 minutes or longer if you prefer. Set a timer if needed to help you stay on track. As you conclude your practice, take a moment to acknowledge the effort you've put in and the benefits you've experienced.

Mindfulness meditation with a focus on the breath is a simple yet profound practice that can have far-reaching effects on your mental, emotional, and physical well-being. By cultivating present-moment awareness and deepening your connection to the breath, you can develop greater clarity, resilience, and inner peace in your life.

CHAPTER 8: Breath and Physical Health

In this chapter, we explore the profound connection between breath and physical health. We delve into the importance of respiratory health and introduce various breathing exercises aimed at improving lung capacity and function.

Respiratory Health and Breathing Exercises

Respiratory health is crucial for overall well-being, as the respiratory system is responsible for supplying oxygen to the body and removing carbon dioxide. Maintaining optimal respiratory health not only ensures efficient oxygenation of tissues but also supports immune function, energy production, and mental clarity. Here, we explore the significance of respiratory health and introduce various breathing exercises aimed at enhancing lung function and promoting overall well-being.

- **Importance of Respiratory Health:**

The respiratory system consists of the airways, lungs, and associated muscles, all working together to facilitate the exchange of gases between the body and the environment.

Healthy respiratory function is essential for:

- **Efficient oxygenation of tissues:** Oxygen is vital for cellular metabolism and energy production in the body. Adequate oxygen supply ensures optimal function of organs and tissues.
- **Removal of carbon dioxide:** The respiratory system eliminates carbon dioxide, a waste product of metabolism, from the body. Proper carbon dioxide removal helps maintain acid-base balance and prevent respiratory acidosis.
- **Immune defense:** The respiratory tract acts as a barrier against pathogens, such as viruses and bacteria, helping to protect the body from respiratory infections.
- **Regulation of pH:** The respiratory system plays a role in regulating blood pH by controlling the levels of carbon dioxide in the bloodstream.

Poor respiratory health can lead to various respiratory conditions, such as asthma, chronic obstructive pulmonary disease (COPD), bronchitis, and pneumonia, as well as symptoms like shortness of breath, coughing, wheezing, and chest tightness.

- **Breathing Exercises for Respiratory Health:**

Incorporating breathing exercises into your daily routine can help strengthen respiratory muscles, improve lung function, and enhance overall respiratory health. Here are some effective breathing exercises to consider:

- **Diaphragmatic Breathing (Deep Belly Breathing):** Diaphragmatic breathing involves engaging the diaphragm muscle to take deep breaths, allowing the abdomen to expand on inhalation and contract on exhalation. This technique helps maximize air exchange, reduce shallow breathing, and promote relaxation.

- **Pursed Lip Breathing:** Pursed lip breathing involves inhaling slowly through the nose and exhaling gently through pursed lips, as if blowing out a candle. This technique helps open up airways, slow down breathing, and improve oxygenation of the blood.

- **Segmental Breathing:** Segmental breathing focuses on expanding and contracting different areas of the lungs sequentially. By directing the breath to specific lung segments, this technique can help improve ventilation and optimize lung function.

- **Box Breathing (Square Breathing):** Box breathing involves inhaling, holding the breath, exhaling, and holding the breath again, each for an equal duration of time. This rhythmic breathing pattern helps calm the nervous system, reduce stress, and enhance respiratory efficiency.

- **Alternate Nostril Breathing (Nadi Shodhana):** Nadi Shodhana is a yogic breathing technique that involves alternating nostrils during inhalation and exhalation. This practice helps balance the flow of prana (life force energy), clear the nasal passages, and promote overall respiratory health.

- **Chest Expansion Exercises:** Chest expansion exercises involve stretching and opening up the chest to improve lung capacity and respiratory function. These exercises may include arm stretches, chest openers, and thoracic spine mobility exercises.

- **Benefits of Breathing Exercises:**

Regular practice of breathing exercises offers numerous benefits for respiratory health and overall well-being, including:

- **Strengthening respiratory muscles**
- **Improving lung function and capacity**
- **Enhancing oxygenation of tissues**
- **Reducing stress and anxiety**
- **Promoting relaxation and men**

Incorporating these breathing exercises into your daily routine can help optimize respiratory function, enhance vitality, and promote a sense of well-being. Remember to practice breathing exercises mindfully and consult with a healthcare professional if you have any underlying respiratory conditions or concerns. With consistent practice and dedication, you can cultivate optimal respiratory health and enjoy the many benefits of mindful breathing.

Improving Lung Capacity and Function

Lung capacity and function play a crucial role in overall respiratory health and physical well-being. Lung capacity refers to the maximum volume of air that the lungs can hold, while lung function refers to how effectively the lungs can exchange oxygen and carbon dioxide. Optimal lung capacity and function are essential for maintaining adequate oxygenation of tissues, supporting physical activity, and preventing respiratory disorders.

Here are some strategies and exercises aimed at improving lung capacity and function:

1. Aerobic Exercise:

Regular aerobic exercise, such as walking, jogging, swimming, cycling, or dancing, can significantly improve lung capacity and function. Aerobic activities increase heart rate and breathing rate, leading to deeper breathing and greater oxygen intake. Over time, aerobic exercise strengthens respiratory muscles, enhances lung elasticity, and improves overall cardiovascular health. Aim for at least 30 minutes of moderate-intensity aerobic exercise most days of the week to reap the benefits for lung capacity and function.

2. Strength Training:

Incorporating strength training exercises into your fitness routine can also benefit lung capacity and function. Strength training exercises, such as weightlifting, resistance band exercises, and bodyweight exercises, help build muscle mass and improve overall strength, including the muscles involved in breathing. Stronger respiratory muscles can generate more forceful contractions, leading to increased lung capacity and improved breathing efficiency.

3. Breathing Exercises:

Specific breathing exercises can target respiratory muscles and enhance lung capacity and function. Some effective breathing exercises include diaphragmatic breathing, pursed lip breathing, segmental breathing, and incentive spirometry. These exercises help strengthen the diaphragm and other respiratory muscles, improve lung ventilation, and optimize breathing mechanics. Practicing breathing exercises regularly can increase lung capacity, improve respiratory endurance, and enhance overall respiratory health.

4. Pulmonary Rehabilitation:

Pulmonary rehabilitation programs are comprehensive interventions designed to improve lung function and quality of life in individuals with chronic respiratory conditions, such as COPD, asthma, and pulmonary fibrosis. These programs typically include exercise training, education, breathing exercises, and psychological support tailored to the individual's needs. Participating in pulmonary rehabilitation can help individuals improve their exercise tolerance, reduce symptoms, and enhance lung function through structured, supervised interventions.

5. Smoking Cessation:

Smoking is a significant risk factor for respiratory diseases and can impair lung function over time. Quitting smoking is one of the most effective ways to improve lung capacity and function and reduce the risk of respiratory disorders. Smoking cessation programs, support groups, and nicotine replacement therapies are available to help individuals quit smoking and improve their respiratory health.

6. Maintaining a Healthy Weight:

Excess body weight can put strain on the respiratory system and decrease lung function. Maintaining a healthy weight through a balanced diet and regular exercise can help optimize lung capacity and function. Losing weight if overweight or obese can improve lung mechanics, reduce respiratory effort, and enhance overall respiratory health.

Improving lung capacity and function requires a multifaceted approach that includes regular exercise, targeted breathing exercises, and lifestyle modifications. By incorporating these strategies into your daily routine, you can enhance respiratory health, increase exercise tolerance, and enjoy a higher quality of life. Remember to consult with a healthcare professional before starting any new exercise program, especially if you have pre-existing respiratory conditions or concerns. With dedication and persistence, you can optimize your lung capacity and function and experience the benefits of improved respiratory health.

CHAPTER 9: Breath and Mental Clarity

In this chapter, we explore the profound connection between breath and mental clarity. We delve into how breathwork can help clear the mind and enhance cognitive function, leading to greater focus, productivity, and overall mental well-being.

Clearing the Mind Through Breath

The breath serves as a bridge between the body and mind, offering a powerful tool for clearing mental clutter, reducing stress, and cultivating a sense of calm and clarity. By bringing attention to the breath and engaging in intentional breathing techniques, individuals can quiet the mind and create space for greater mental clarity.
Here's how breathwork can help clear the mind:

1. Deep Breathing:

Deep breathing exercises, such as diaphragmatic breathing or belly breathing, involve taking slow, deliberate breaths that fully engage the diaphragm. By expanding the lungs to their full capacity and exhaling slowly and completely, individuals can activate the body's relaxation response, calm the nervous system, and quiet mental chatter.

2. Mindful Breathing:

Mindful breathing involves bringing full awareness to each breath as it enters and leaves the body. By observing the sensations of the breath without judgment or attachment, individuals can anchor their attention in the present moment and cultivate a sense of mindfulness. Mindful breathing allows individuals to let go of distractions and worries, returning to the here and now with greater clarity and focus.

3. Breath Awareness Meditation:

Breath awareness meditation is a practice of focusing solely on the breath as a meditation object. By directing attention to the rhythmic flow of the breath, individuals can train the mind to become more centered and attentive. As thoughts and distractions arise, individuals gently guide their attention back to the breath, cultivating a sense of inner calm and clarity.

4. Breath Counting:

Breath counting is a simple yet effective technique for clearing the mind. Individuals count each inhalation and exhalation, starting from one and continuing up to a predetermined number, such as ten. By focusing on the rhythmic counting of breaths, individuals can quiet mental distractions and cultivate greater concentration and presence.

5. Paced Breathing:

Paced breathing involves regulating the breath to a specific rhythm or cadence. By synchronizing the breath with a counting pattern, individuals can induce a state of relaxation and mental clarity. Paced breathing techniques, such as box breathing or resonant breathing, help balance the autonomic nervous system, reduce stress, and promote a sense of well-being.

6. Breathwork Practices:

Various breathwork practices, such as pranayama in yoga or qigong breathing exercises, offer additional tools for clearing the mind. These practices involve specific breathing patterns and techniques aimed at harmonizing the body, mind, and spirit. By engaging in breathwork practices, individuals can release tension, quiet the mind, and access deeper states of relaxation and awareness.

Clearing the mind through breath requires patience, practice, and consistent effort. By incorporating breathwork techniques into daily life, individuals can cultivate greater mental clarity, resilience, and well-being. Whether used as a standalone practice or integrated into meditation and mindfulness routines, breathwork offers a valuable pathway to inner peace and clarity of mind.

Breathwork for Enhanced Cognitive Function

Breathwork techniques offer a powerful means of enhancing cognitive function, sharpening mental acuity, and optimizing overall brain health. By regulating the breath and increasing oxygenation to the brain, individuals can boost cognitive performance, improve focus, and enhance mental clarity. Here's how breathwork can contribute to enhanced cognitive function:

1. Box Breathing:

Box breathing, also known as square breathing, is a simple yet effective technique for enhancing cognitive function. This technique involves inhaling, holding the breath, exhaling, and holding the breath again, each for equal counts. By regulating the breath in this rhythmic pattern, individuals can balance the autonomic nervous system, reduce stress, and promote mental focus and clarity.

2. Alternate Nostril Breathing (Nadi Shodhana):

Nadi Shodhana, or alternate nostril breathing, is a yogic breathing technique that helps balance the flow of prana (life force energy) and clear the mind. This practice involves alternating nostrils during inhalation and exhalation, using the thumb and ring finger to block one nostril at a time. Nadi Shodhana helps synchronize the hemispheres of the brain, promote mental balance, and enhance cognitive function.

3. Brain Wave Entrainment:

Certain breathwork techniques, such as rhythmic breathing or coherent breathing, can entrain brain wave patterns and induce a state of mental coherence. By synchronizing brain waves to specific frequencies, individuals can optimize cognitive function, enhance creativity, and improve overall brain health. Brain wave entrainment techniques can be achieved through guided breathwork exercises or specialized audio recordings.

4. Breath Retention (Kumbhaka):

Breath retention practices involve holding the breath for extended periods, either after inhalation (antara kumbhaka) or after exhalation (bahya kumbhaka). These practices stimulate the vagus nerve, increase cerebral blood flow, and improve oxygenation to the brain. By incorporating breath retention into their practice, individuals can enhance mental clarity, concentration, and cognitive performance.

5. Pranayama:

Pranayama, or yogic breath control, encompasses a wide range of techniques for regulating the breath and cultivating energy and awareness. Practices such as Kapalabhati (skull-shining breath) or Bhastrika (bellows breath) involve rapid, forceful breathing patterns that increase oxygen intake and activate the sympathetic nervous system. These practices help sharpen mental acuity, increase alertness, and optimize cognitive function.

6. Mindful Breathing:

Mindful breathing practices, such as breath awareness meditation or mindful breathing exercises, can also enhance cognitive function. By bringing full awareness to each breath and observing the sensations without judgment or attachment, individuals can cultivate present-moment awareness and mental clarity. Mindful breathing helps quiet the mind, reduce distractions, and improve cognitive performance.

By incorporating breathwork techniques into daily life, individuals can optimize cognitive function, enhance mental clarity, and support overall brain health. Whether used as a standalone practice or integrated into meditation and mindfulness routines, breathwork offers a valuable tool for unlocking the full potential of the mind and promoting cognitive well-being.

CHAPTER 10: Holistic Healing with Breath

In this chapter, we explore the profound role of breath in holistic healing practices. We delve into how breathwork can facilitate energy healing and integration into various holistic health modalities, fostering overall well-being and vitality.

Breathwork and Energy Healing

Breathwork is deeply intertwined with energy healing practices across various cultures and traditions, offering a profound pathway for accessing and channeling vital life force energy. This synergy between breath and energy lies at the heart of many holistic healing modalities, facilitating balance, restoration, and transformation on physical, emotional, mental, and spiritual levels.

Here's how breathwork contributes to energy healing:

- **Prana, Qi, and Life Force Energy:**

In traditional healing systems such as yoga, Ayurveda, and Traditional Chinese Medicine (TCM), there is a recognition of a vital life force energy that animates all living beings.

Known as prana in yoga, qi in TCM, or simply life force energy, this subtle energy is believed to flow through the body's energy channels (nadis in yoga, meridians in TCM), nourishing and sustaining every aspect of our being.

Breathwork serves as a direct means of accessing and cultivating this life force energy. Through conscious regulation of the breath, individuals can enhance the flow of prana or qi within the body, clear energetic blockages, and restore harmony to the energy system. This facilitates holistic healing and supports overall well-being.

- **Chakra Activation:**

The chakras are energy centers located along the spine, each associated with specific physical, emotional, and spiritual aspects of our being. Breathwork techniques can activate and balance the chakras, promoting energetic alignment and facilitating healing on multiple levels.

Various breathwork practices, such as visualization, sound, and specific breathing patterns, can stimulate and harmonize the chakras. For example, focused breathing on specific energy centers or using specific mantras associated with each chakra can help awaken and balance the corresponding chakra, promoting overall energy flow and vitality.

- **Breath of Fire (Kapalabhati) and Dynamic Breathwork:**

Breath of Fire, a dynamic breathing technique in yoga, involves rapid, rhythmic breathing through the nose. This powerful practice increases prana flow, clears stagnant energy, and awakens the body's natural healing abilities. Similarly, other forms of dynamic breathwork, such as Holotropic Breathwork or Rebirthing Breathwork, utilize intense breathing patterns to facilitate altered states of consciousness, emotional release, and spiritual awakening.

These dynamic breathwork practices can induce profound shifts in energy, helping individuals release stored tension, trauma, and emotional blockages. By accessing deeper layers of consciousness and connecting with the innate wisdom of the body, individuals can experience profound healing and transformation.

- **Breathwork Integration in Energy Healing Modalities:**

Breathwork is often integrated into various energy healing modalities, enhancing their effectiveness and supporting holistic healing. For example, breathwork may be incorporated into Reiki sessions to deepen relaxation, increase energy flow, and facilitate emotional release. Similarly, in acupuncture or acupressure sessions, conscious breathing techniques can help individuals release tension and amplify the effects of the treatment.

Breathwork may also be used in conjunction with other energy healing practices, such as crystal healing, sound therapy, or shamanic healing, to enhance energetic resonance and promote balance and harmony in the body-mind-spirit system.

By embracing the synergy between breathwork and energy healing, individuals can access the transformative power of breath to promote healing, balance, and vitality on all levels of their being. Whether used as a standalone practice or integrated into other holistic healing modalities, breathwork offers a profound pathway for connecting with our innate healing potential and embracing the fullness of our being.

Integrating Breath into Holistic Health Practices

Breathwork serves as a foundational component of holistic health practices, offering a versatile and accessible tool for promoting well-being on physical, emotional, mental, and spiritual levels. By integrating breathwork into holistic health modalities, individuals can enhance their effectiveness, deepen their healing potential, and cultivate greater harmony and balance in their lives. Here's how breath can be integrated into various holistic health practices:

1. Mindfulness-Based Stress Reduction (MBSR):

Mindfulness-based stress reduction programs often incorporate breath awareness and mindful breathing practices as core components. By cultivating present-moment awareness and nonjudgmental acceptance of the breath, individuals can reduce stress, enhance resilience, and improve overall well-being. Breath-focused meditation, body scan exercises, and mindful movement practices can help individuals develop greater mindfulness and self-awareness.

2. Yoga and Meditation:

Yoga and meditation practices traditionally include breathwork techniques, known as pranayama, as an integral part of their practice. By coordinating movement with breath and cultivating breath awareness, individuals can deepen their yoga and meditation practices, quiet the mind, and connect with their inner wisdom. Pranayama techniques such as deep belly breathing, alternate nostril breathing, and breath retention can help regulate the nervous system, balance energy, and promote holistic health.

3. Body-Mind Therapies:

Body-mind therapies, such as somatic experiencing, breathwork therapy, and integrative bodywork, often incorporate breath awareness and conscious breathing techniques to facilitate healing on physical, emotional, and energetic levels. These therapies help individuals release tension, trauma, and holding patterns stored in the body, promoting holistic healing and integration. Breath-focused interventions, such as guided imagery, progressive relaxation, and breath-based movement practices, can support clients in accessing and processing unresolved emotions and experiences.

4. Energy Medicine:

Energy medicine modalities, such as acupuncture, acupressure, and energy healing, work with the body's subtle energy systems to promote balance and well-being. Breathwork can enhance the effectiveness of energy medicine practices by facilitating the flow of prana or qi, supporting the body's natural healing processes, and restoring energetic harmony. Conscious breathing techniques may be integrated into energy healing sessions to deepen relaxation, enhance energy flow, and promote emotional release and energetic clearing.

5. Holistic Psychotherapy:

Holistic psychotherapy approaches, such as transpersonal therapy, integrative psychotherapy, and breathwork-oriented psychotherapy, incorporate breath awareness and conscious breathing techniques to support emotional healing, self-exploration, and personal growth. These approaches help individuals access deeper layers of consciousness, process unresolved emotions, and integrate body, mind, and spirit. Breath-focused interventions, such as breathwork exercises, guided imagery, and breath-centered mindfulness practices, can facilitate the exploration and resolution of psychological issues and promote holistic well-being.

6. Daily Self-Care Practices:

Incorporating breathwork into daily self-care practices can also support holistic health and well-being. Simple breath awareness exercises, such as taking a few mindful breaths before meals or pausing to notice the breath during moments of stress, can help individuals cultivate greater presence, relaxation, and inner peace. Regular breathwork routines, such as morning breathing exercises or evening relaxation practices, can serve as anchors for self-care and resilience-building, fostering a deeper connection with oneself and promoting overall vitality and balance.

By integrating breathwork into holistic health practices, individuals can harness the transformative power of the breath to support their journey toward greater health, healing, and wholeness. Whether used as a standalone practice or combined with other modalities, breathwork offers a versatile and accessible tool for cultivating well-being on all levels of the body-mind-spirit system.

CHAPTER 11: Breath and Sleep

In this chapter, we explore the intricate relationship between breath and sleep, focusing on how specific breath techniques can enhance sleep quality and address common sleep disorders. By harnessing the power of breath, individuals can cultivate better sleep patterns and improve overall well-being.

Breath Techniques for Better Sleep

Sleep is essential for overall health and well-being, yet many people struggle with falling asleep or staying asleep throughout the night. Incorporating breath techniques into your bedtime routine can help calm the mind, relax the body, and facilitate a smoother transition into restful sleep. Here are some effective breath techniques for better sleep:

1. Deep Belly Breathing:
Deep belly breathing, also known as diaphragmatic breathing, involves breathing deeply into the abdomen, allowing the diaphragm to fully expand and contract with each breath.

To practice deep belly breathing:

- Find a comfortable lying position in bed.
- Place one hand on your abdomen and the other on your chest.
- Inhale deeply through your nose, allowing your abdomen to rise as you fill your lungs with air.
- Exhale slowly and completely through your mouth, feeling your abdomen fall as you release the breath.
- Continue breathing deeply and rhythmically, focusing on the sensation of your breath moving in and out of your body.

Deep belly breathing activates the body's relaxation response, reduces stress hormones, and promotes a sense of calm conducive to sleep.

2. 4-7-8 Breathing:

The 4-7-8 breathing technique is a simple yet powerful method for inducing relaxation and promoting better sleep. To practice 4-7-8 breathing:

- Begin by exhaling completely through your mouth, making a whooshing sound.

- Close your mouth and inhale silently through your nose for a count of 4.
- Hold your breath for a count of 7.
- Exhale slowly and completely through your mouth for a count of 8, making a whooshing sound.
- Repeat this cycle for several rounds, focusing on the rhythmic pattern of your breath.

4-7-8 breathing helps regulate the autonomic nervous system, calm the mind, and induce a state of relaxation conducive to sleep.

3. Nadi Shodhana (Alternate Nostril Breathing):
Nadi Shodhana, a yogic breathing technique, helps balance the flow of energy in the body, calm the mind, and promote mental clarity.
To practice Nadi Shodhana:

- Sit comfortably with your spine straight and shoulders relaxed.
- Close your right nostril with your right thumb and inhale slowly and deeply through your left nostril.
- Close your left nostril with your right ring finger and exhale through your right nostril.

- Inhale through your right nostril, then close it with your right thumb and exhale through your left nostril.

- Continue this alternating pattern of inhaling and exhaling through each nostril for several rounds, maintaining a slow and steady pace.

Nadi Shodhana helps quiet the mind, balance the nervous system, and promote a sense of inner peace conducive to sleep.

4. Progressive Muscle Relaxation with Breath:

Progressive muscle relaxation involves systematically tensing and relaxing different muscle groups in the body to release tension and promote relaxation. Combining progressive muscle relaxation with breathwork can enhance its effectiveness for better sleep.

To practice progressive muscle relaxation with breath:

- Start by lying comfortably in bed and taking a few deep breaths to center yourself.

- Begin with your toes, tensing them tightly for a few seconds, then releasing and relaxing them completely as you exhale.

- Continue this process, moving upward through each muscle group in your body, including your calves,

thighs, buttocks, abdomen, chest, arms, shoulders, neck, and face.

- With each exhalation, imagine tension melting away from your muscles, leaving you feeling deeply relaxed and at ease.

Progressive muscle relaxation with breath helps release physical tension, quiet the mind, and prepare the body for sleep.

Incorporating these breath techniques into your bedtime routine can help calm the nervous system, reduce stress, and promote a sense of relaxation conducive to better sleep. Experiment with different techniques to find what works best for you, and make breathwork a regular part of your sleep hygiene practices for improved sleep quality and overall well-being.

Addressing Sleep Disorders Through Breath

Sleep disorders such as insomnia, sleep apnea, and restless leg syndrome can significantly impact an individual's quality of life, affecting their physical health, cognitive function, and emotional well-being. Fortunately, breathwork techniques offer a natural and accessible approach to addressing these sleep disturbances, promoting relaxation, regulating the nervous system, and improving overall sleep quality. Here's how breathwork can help address common sleep disorders:

Insomnia:

Insomnia is characterized by difficulty falling asleep or staying asleep, often resulting in daytime fatigue, irritability, and impaired cognitive function. Breathwork techniques can help individuals with insomnia calm the mind, reduce anxiety, and create a conducive environment for sleep. Here's how breathwork can address insomnia:

- **Deep Belly Breathing:** Practicing deep belly breathing before bedtime activates the body's relaxation response, reduces stress hormones, and promotes a sense of calm conducive to sleep initiation.

- **4-7-8 Breathing:** The 4-7-8 breathing technique helps regulate the autonomic nervous system, induce relaxation, and quiet the mind, making it easier to fall asleep and stay asleep throughout the night.

- **Mindful Breathing:** Mindful breathing practices involve bringing full awareness to each breath as it enters and leaves the body, helping individuals let go of racing thoughts and worries that may interfere with sleep.

By incorporating these breathwork techniques into their bedtime routine, individuals with insomnia can promote relaxation, reduce sleep latency, and improve overall sleep quality.

Sleep Apnea:

Sleep apnea is a sleep disorder characterized by interruptions in breathing during sleep, leading to fragmented sleep, daytime sleepiness, and increased risk of cardiovascular problems. Breathwork techniques can help individuals with sleep apnea improve breathing patterns, reduce the frequency of apneic episodes, and promote better sleep quality.

Here's how breathwork can address sleep apnea:

- **Diaphragmatic Breathing:** Diaphragmatic breathing strengthens the respiratory muscles, improves lung capacity, and promotes proper breathing mechanics, reducing the likelihood of obstructive events during sleep.

- **Box Breathing:** Box breathing involves inhaling, holding the breath, exhaling, and holding the breath again, each for equal counts. This rhythmic breathing pattern helps regulate breathing and reduce respiratory irregularities during sleep.

- **Pranayama Techniques:** Pranayama techniques such as Kapalabhati (skull-shining breath) and Bhastrika (bellows breath) can increase oxygenation, enhance respiratory function, and reduce the severity of sleep apnea symptoms.

By incorporating these breathwork techniques into their daily routine, individuals with sleep apnea can improve respiratory function, reduce sleep disturbances, and enhance overall sleep quality.

Restless Leg Syndrome (RLS):

Restless leg syndrome (RLS) is a neurological disorder characterized by uncomfortable sensations in the legs, often accompanied by an irresistible urge to move the legs, especially at night. Breathwork techniques can help individuals with RLS alleviate symptoms, reduce muscle tension, and promote relaxation conducive to sleep. Here's how breathwork can address RLS:

- 4-7-8 Breathing: The 4-7-8 breathing technique induces relaxation, calms the nervous system, and reduces muscle tension, helping individuals with RLS ease discomfort and promote restful sleep.

- Progressive Muscle Relaxation with Breath: Progressive muscle relaxation combined with deep breathing can help individuals with RLS release physical tension, alleviate symptoms, and prepare the body for sleep.

- Mindfulness Meditation: Mindfulness meditation with breath focus can help individuals with RLS cultivate present-moment awareness, reduce anxiety, and promote acceptance of discomfort, making it easier to cope with symptoms and fall asleep.

By practicing these breathwork techniques regularly, individuals with RLS can reduce symptom severity, improve sleep quality, and enhance overall well-being.

Incorporating breathwork techniques into a comprehensive sleep hygiene routine can be a valuable tool for managing sleep disorders and promoting better sleep quality. Whether used alone or in conjunction with other treatment modalities, breathwork offers a natural and effective approach to addressing the underlying factors contributing to sleep disturbances, restoring balance to the body-mind system, and fostering a deeper sense of relaxation and well-being.

CHAPTER 12: Breath in Movement

In this chapter, we explore the importance of integrating breath into movement practices, such as exercise, physical activity, and yoga. By consciously coordinating breath with movement, individuals can enhance performance, improve body awareness, and cultivate a deeper sense of connection between mind, body, and breath.

Integrating Breath into Exercise and Physical Activity

Breath is a fundamental component of movement, influencing both performance and overall well-being during exercise and physical activity. By understanding how to synchronize breath with movement, individuals can optimize their performance, enhance endurance, and reduce the risk of injury. Here's how to effectively integrate breath into exercise and physical activity:

1. Synchronize Breath with Movement:

One of the key principles of integrating breath into exercise is synchronizing breath with movement. The goal is to coordinate inhalation and exhalation with specific phases of movement to maximize efficiency and effectiveness. Here's a general guideline:

- **Inhalation:** Inhale during the preparatory phase or the "easy" part of the movement. For example, when lowering into a squat or extending the arms overhead.

- **Exhalation:** Exhale during the exertion or the "hard" part of the movement. This includes phases such as lifting a weight, pushing off the ground during a jump, or rising from a squat.

By synchronizing breath with movement, individuals can enhance stability, control, and power output, leading to improved performance and reduced strain on the body.

2. Use Breath to Manage Intensity:

Breath can also be used as a tool for managing intensity during exercise. Deepening the breath during challenging moments can help individuals stay focused, calm, and resilient in the face of physical exertion. This is particularly beneficial during high-intensity intervals, strength training sets, or endurance activities.

- **Deep Breathing:** Taking deep, diaphragmatic breaths can help oxygenate the body, reduce muscle tension, and promote relaxation during intense exercise. Inhale deeply through the nose, allowing the abdomen to expand, and exhale fully through the mouth, releasing tension and fatigue.

- **Controlled Breathing:** Consciously controlling the pace and depth of breathing can help regulate heart rate and prevent hyperventilation during intense exercise. Individuals can experiment with different breathing patterns, such as inhaling for a certain count and exhaling for a longer count, to find what works best for them.

3. Maintain Consistent Breathing Patterns:

Consistency in breathing patterns is essential for optimizing energy flow and efficiency during exercise. Whether performing repetitive movements or dynamic sequences, maintaining a steady rhythm of breath helps regulate heart rate, improve oxygen uptake, and promote a state of flow and concentration.

- **Rhythmic Breathing:** Establishing a rhythm of breath that matches the cadence of movement can help create a sense of flow and synchronicity during exercise. For example, in running or cycling, individuals may synchronize their breath with their stride or pedal cadence to maintain a steady pace and conserve energy.

By incorporating these principles into their exercise routine, individuals can harness the power of breath to enhance performance, improve endurance, and deepen their mind-body connection during physical activity. Whether engaging in cardio exercises, strength training, or flexibility routines, integrating breath into movement can optimize results and promote overall well-being.

Yoga and Breath-Centric Movement

Yoga is a holistic practice that emphasizes the integration of breath with movement, fostering a deep connection between mind, body, and breath. Breath-centric movement, commonly known as vinyasa or flow, is a cornerstone of yoga practice, promoting flexibility, strength, balance, and inner awareness. Here's how yoga incorporates breath into movement:

1. Linking Breath with Movement:

In yoga, each movement is synchronized with either an inhalation or an exhalation, creating a seamless flow of breath and movement. This rhythmic synchronization helps individuals cultivate mindfulness, focus, and presence throughout their practice.
For example:

- **Inhale:** Inhalation is often associated with movements that open the body, such as extending the arms overhead or lifting the chest in a backbend.
- **Exhale:** Exhalation is typically linked with movements that contract or fold the body, such as folding forward or twisting to one side.

By linking breath with movement, individuals can move more mindfully, deepen their stretches, and cultivate a meditative state of awareness on the mat.

2. Ujjayi Breathing:

Ujjayi breath, also known as "ocean breath" or "victorious breath," is a foundational pranayama technique used in yoga to regulate the breath and create internal heat. Practiced by slightly constricting the back of the throat, Ujjayi breath produces a gentle whispering sound with each inhalation and exhalation. This audible breath helps individuals deepen their breath awareness, enhance concentration, and maintain a steady rhythm throughout their practice.

3. Breath Awareness in Asana Practice:

Beyond vinyasa sequences, yoga emphasizes breath awareness in static asanas (poses) as well. Individuals are encouraged to maintain smooth, steady breaths throughout each pose, using the breath as a tool for deepening the stretch, releasing tension, and accessing deeper layers of awareness. For example:

- In forward folds, individuals can exhale deeply to release tension in the hamstrings and spine, allowing for a deeper stretch.
- In backbends, individuals can inhale fully to expand the chest and lift the heart, creating space in the front body while maintaining stability and support.

By focusing on breath awareness in asana practice, individuals can cultivate a greater sense of presence, mindfulness, and inner calm, both on and off the mat.

Yoga's emphasis on breath-centric movement extends beyond the physical postures, influencing all aspects of the practice, including meditation, chanting, and relaxation techniques. By integrating breath with movement, yoga offers a holistic pathway for individuals to cultivate strength, flexibility, and inner peace, fostering a deeper connection with themselves and the world around them. Whether practicing a vigorous vinyasa flow or a gentle restorative sequence, the breath remains a constant anchor, guiding individuals back to the present moment and the essence of yoga: union of body, mind, and breath.

CHAPTER 13: Breath in Daily Life

In this chapter, we explore the practical application of breath techniques in everyday situations, offering strategies for managing stress, promoting relaxation, and enhancing well-being through on-the-go breathing practices.

Applying Breath Techniques in Everyday Situations

Breath techniques offer practical and accessible ways to manage stress, enhance focus, and promote relaxation in various everyday situations. By incorporating simple breath practices into daily routines, individuals can cultivate mindfulness, reduce anxiety, and improve overall well-being. Here are some ways to apply breath techniques in everyday situations:

- **Workplace:**

- **Desk Breathing:** Take short breaks throughout the workday to practice deep breathing at your desk. Close your eyes, inhale deeply through your nose, and exhale slowly through your mouth. This can help alleviate tension, increase oxygen flow to the brain, and improve focus and productivity.

- **Meeting Preparation:** Before important meetings or presentations, take a few moments to practice calming breath techniques such as 4-7-8 breathing or diaphragmatic breathing. This can help reduce nervousness, boost confidence, and improve clarity of thought.

- **Commute:**

- **Traffic Stress Relief:** Use your commute time as an opportunity to practice mindfulness and relaxation. Focus on your breath while stuck in traffic or waiting for public transportation. Inhale deeply through your nose, exhale slowly through your mouth, and let go of tension with each breath.

- **Mindful Walking:** If you walk or bike to work, incorporate mindful breathing into your commute. Pay attention to the rhythm of your breath as you move, feeling the sensation of air entering and leaving your body with each step or pedal.

- **Daily Routine:**

- **Morning Ritual:** Start your day with a few minutes of mindful breathing before getting out of bed. Inhale deeply, feeling your chest and abdomen expand, and exhale slowly, releasing any tension or stress from the previous day. This can set a positive tone for the day ahead.

- **Mealtime Mindfulness:** Practice mindful eating by taking a few deep breaths before each meal. This can help you tune into your body's hunger and fullness cues, savor the flavors of your food, and promote digestion and relaxation.

- **Social Interactions:**

- **Pre-Event Preparation:** Before social events or gatherings, take a moment to practice calming breath techniques to reduce anxiety and nervousness. Inhale deeply to center yourself, exhale slowly to release tension, and approach social interactions with a sense of calm and presence.

- **Active Listening:** During conversations with others, practice mindful breathing to stay present and attentive.

Focus on your breath while listening to the speaker, allowing yourself to fully engage in the conversation without distraction or judgment.

Incorporating breath techniques into everyday situations doesn't require extra time or special equipment, making it a convenient and effective way to promote well-being throughout the day. By cultivating mindfulness and relaxation through breath practices, individuals can navigate daily challenges with greater ease, resilience, and inner peace.

Managing Stress with On-the-Go Breathing Practices

In our fast-paced lives, stress can often feel unavoidable. However, incorporating on-the-go breathing practices into daily routines can provide a simple yet effective way to manage stress and promote relaxation, even amidst busy schedules and demanding situations. Here are some portable breath techniques that can be practiced anytime, anywhere:

1. Square Breathing (Box Breathing):

Square breathing is a technique that involves inhaling, holding the breath, exhaling, and holding the breath again, each for an equal count of seconds. This simple and systematic approach can quickly calm the nervous system and promote a sense of balance and tranquility. Here's how to practice square breathing:

- Inhale deeply through the nose for a count of four.
- Hold the breath at the top of the inhale for a count of four.
- Exhale slowly and completely through the mouth for a count of four.
- Hold the breath at the bottom of the exhale for a count of four.
- Repeat this cycle for several rounds, focusing on the rhythmic pattern of breath.

2. Counted Breaths:

Counting breaths involves inhaling slowly and deeply through the nose for a specific count, holding the breath briefly, and then exhaling slowly and completely through the mouth for the same count. This technique helps regulate breathing patterns, promote relaxation, and reduce tension in the body and mind. Here's how to practice counted breaths:

- Inhale deeply through the nose for a count of four.
- Hold the breath at the top of the inhale for a count of four.
- Exhale slowly and completely through the mouth for a count of four.
- Repeat this cycle for several rounds, maintaining a steady and even pace of breath.

3. Mindful Breathing:

Mindful breathing involves bringing full awareness to each breath as it enters and leaves the body, without judgment or attachment. This practice can help individuals cultivate mindfulness, reduce stress, and promote a sense of inner peace. Here's how to practice mindful breathing:

- Find a comfortable seated or standing position.
- Close your eyes or soften your gaze.
- Focus your attention on the sensation of your breath as it moves in and out of your body.
- Notice the rise and fall of your chest or abdomen with each inhale and exhale.

- If your mind wanders, gently bring your attention back to the breath without judgment.

4. Quick Reset Breath:

The quick reset breath is a technique that involves taking a deep breath in through the nose, holding it for a moment, and then exhaling forcefully through the mouth with a sigh or audible sound. This quick burst of breath can help release tension, reset the nervous system, and promote relaxation in stressful situations. Here's how to practice the quick reset breath:

- Inhale deeply through the nose, filling your lungs with air.
- Hold the breath for a moment at the top of the inhale.
- Exhale forcefully through the mouth with a sigh or audible sound, letting go of any tension or stress.
- Repeat this cycle as needed to help restore a sense of calm and balance.

Incorporating these on-the-go breathing practices into daily routines can provide individuals with valuable tools for managing stress, promoting relaxation, and enhancing overall well-being. Whether practiced during commutes, work breaks, or moments of downtime, breath techniques offer a simple yet powerful way to cultivate mindfulness and resilience in the face of life's challenges.

CHAPTER 14: Breath and Emotional Well-being

In this chapter, we delve into the profound connection between breath and emotional well-being, exploring how breathwork techniques can be used for emotional regulation and how expressive arts can deepen this connection.

Breathwork for Emotional Regulation

Breathwork techniques offer powerful tools for emotional regulation, providing individuals with practical methods to manage and navigate their emotions effectively. By consciously engaging with the breath, individuals can influence their physiological and psychological states, fostering greater emotional balance, resilience, and well-being. Here are some breathwork practices commonly used for emotional regulation:

1. Calm Abiding Breath (Mindfulness Breathing):

Calm abiding breath, also known as mindfulness breathing, involves observing the natural flow of the breath without attempting to control or manipulate it. This practice encourages individuals to anchor their awareness in the present moment, cultivating a sense of calm and centeredness. By focusing on the sensations of the breath as it enters and leaves the body, individuals can develop greater emotional resilience and non-reactivity to challenging emotions.

2. Emotional Release Breath:

Emotional release breathwork involves using the breath to release pent-up emotions and tension held in the body. Through deep, rhythmic breathing, individuals can access and express suppressed emotions, allowing for greater emotional freedom and catharsis. This practice may involve consciously breathing into areas of the body where emotions are felt most intensely, such as the chest or abdomen, and allowing the breath to facilitate the release of emotional energy.

3. Heart-Centered Breath:

Heart-centered breathwork focuses on breathing into the heart center, fostering feelings of compassion, empathy, and connection with oneself and others. This practice encourages individuals to cultivate a sense of warmth and acceptance towards their emotions, allowing them to be fully present with whatever arises. By breathing into the heart space, individuals can access a deeper sense of emotional openness, vulnerability, and authenticity.

4. Alternate Nostril Breathing (Nadi Shodhana):

Alternate nostril breathing, or Nadi Shodhana, is a pranayama technique that involves alternating the breath between the left and right nostrils. This practice helps balance the flow of energy in the body, harmonize the nervous system, and promote emotional equilibrium. By regulating the breath through alternate nostril breathing, individuals can calm the mind, reduce anxiety, and enhance emotional stability.

5. Box Breathing:

Box breathing is a simple yet effective breathwork technique that involves inhaling, holding the breath, exhaling, and holding the breath again, each for an equal count of seconds. This rhythmic breathing pattern helps regulate the autonomic nervous system, induce relaxation, and reduce emotional reactivity. By practicing box breathing, individuals can create a sense of spaciousness and ease in the mind and body, allowing for greater emotional clarity and self-awareness.

Incorporating these breathwork practices into daily life can provide individuals with valuable tools for managing stress, regulating emotions, and promoting overall emotional well-being. Whether practiced as a standalone activity or integrated into other mindfulness or self-care practices, breathwork offers a pathway to greater emotional resilience, balance, and harmony.

Expressive Arts and Breath Connection

The expressive arts provide a unique and powerful avenue for exploring the connection between breath and emotional expression, creativity, and healing. By integrating breathwork techniques with various artistic modalities, individuals can deepen their self-awareness, access deeper layers of emotion, and promote holistic well-being. Here's how expressive arts practices can enhance the breath-emotion connection:

1. Breath-Inspired Movement:

Movement-based expressive arts practices, such as dance, yoga, tai chi, and qigong, integrate breath with movement to promote emotional expression, release, and integration. By syncing breath with movement, individuals can access embodied wisdom, release physical and emotional tension, and cultivate a greater sense of connection with themselves and others. Breath-inspired movement allows for the expression of emotions that may be difficult to articulate verbally, providing a non-verbal outlet for emotional release and healing.

2. Breathwork in Visual Arts:

Visual arts practices, such as painting, drawing, and sculpture, can be enhanced by incorporating breathwork techniques. By consciously connecting with the breath while creating art, individuals can tap into their intuition, creativity, and emotional depth. Breath-driven art-making allows for a spontaneous and authentic expression of emotions, providing a safe and supportive space for exploring and processing complex feelings. Through the act of creation, individuals can externalize and transform their innermost thoughts and emotions into tangible works of art.

3. Breath-Informed Music and Sound:

Music and sound-based expressive arts practices, such as singing, chanting, playing musical instruments, and sound healing, can be enriched by conscious breathing techniques. By synchronizing breath with sound production, individuals can amplify the emotional resonance of their music, deepen their connection with the music-making process, and access profound states of emotional catharsis and healing. Breath-informed music and sound offer a powerful vehicle for emotional expression, communication, and connection, transcending language and cultural barriers.

4. Breath-Based Writing and Poetry:

Writing and poetry can also be informed by breathwork techniques, allowing individuals to tap into their creative flow and emotional depth. By connecting with the breath while writing, individuals can access a state of relaxed focus, flow, and inspiration. Breath-based writing and poetry provide a means of expressing and processing complex emotions, gaining insights into one's inner world, and fostering greater self-awareness and self-expression. Through the rhythmic interplay of breath and language, individuals can create poetry and prose that resonate with authenticity, depth, and emotional resonance.

Incorporating breathwork techniques into expressive arts practices offers a holistic approach to emotional expression, creativity, and healing. By engaging with the breath through movement, visual arts, music, sound, writing, and poetry, individuals can access deeper layers of emotion, creativity, and self-discovery, fostering greater emotional well-being, resilience, and fulfillment. Whether practiced individually or in a group setting, expressive arts and breath connection provide a powerful pathway to self-expression, transformation, and wholeness.

CHAPTER 15: Breath as a Tool for Self-Discovery

In this chapter, we delve into the transformative potential of breath as a tool for self-discovery, exploring how breathwork techniques can facilitate personal growth, self-reflection, and inner exploration.

Exploring Personal Growth Through Breath

Breathwork offers a profound pathway for personal growth and self-discovery, providing individuals with the opportunity to delve deeply into their inner landscape, uncovering insights, and fostering transformative change. Here's how exploring personal growth through breath can unfold:

1. Connecting with Inner Wisdom:

One of the most powerful aspects of breathwork is its ability to quiet the mind and connect individuals with their inner wisdom and intuition. Through practices such as mindfulness breathing or deep relaxation, individuals can create a space of stillness and receptivity, allowing insights and guidance to arise naturally. By tuning into the rhythm of their breath, individuals can access a deeper level of consciousness where answers to life's questions may become clearer.

2. Releasing Limiting Beliefs:

Breathwork can serve as a catalyst for identifying and releasing limiting beliefs, fears, and patterns that may be holding individuals back from reaching their full potential. As individuals bring awareness to their breath and allow it to penetrate areas of tension and resistance in the body, they may encounter emotional blockages that have been stored within them. Through continued breathwork practice, individuals can gently release these energetic blockages, allowing for greater freedom, empowerment, and personal growth.

3. Cultivating Presence and Mindfulness:

Engaging in breathwork encourages individuals to cultivate presence and mindfulness in their daily lives. By anchoring their awareness in the present moment through the breath, individuals can develop a greater capacity to fully engage with each experience with openness and curiosity. This heightened state of awareness fosters resilience, acceptance, and appreciation for the richness of life's experiences, ultimately leading to personal growth and self-actualization.

4. Embracing Vulnerability and Authenticity:

Breathwork provides a safe and supportive container for individuals to explore their vulnerabilities and embrace their authenticity. As individuals surrender to the rhythmic flow of their breath, they may find themselves opening up to deeper layers of emotion and self-expression. Through this process of self-discovery, individuals can cultivate greater self-acceptance, self-love, and compassion, paving the way for profound personal growth and transformation.

5. Integrating Insights into Daily Life:

The insights gained through breathwork practice can be integrated into daily life, serving as guideposts for personal growth and evolution. Whether it's recognizing patterns of behavior that no longer serve them, setting intentions for positive change, or embodying newfound insights and wisdom, individuals can apply the lessons learned from breathwork to all aspects of their lives, leading to greater fulfillment, resilience, and well-being.

In summary, exploring personal growth through breath offers a transformative journey of self-discovery, empowerment, and healing. By engaging in breathwork practices with openness, curiosity, and intention, individuals can connect with their inner wisdom, release what no longer serves them, and embrace their authentic selves, ultimately leading to profound personal growth and transformation.

Using Breathwork for Self-Reflection

Breathwork serves as a powerful tool for self-reflection, providing individuals with a means to explore their inner landscape, gain insight into their thoughts and emotions, and foster personal growth and transformation. Here's how breathwork can be used for self-reflection:

1. Journaling and Breath Awareness:

Pairing breathwork practices with journaling enhances self-reflection and deepens insight. After a breathwork session, individuals can take time to write about their experiences, thoughts, and emotions. By journaling, individuals can gain clarity and perspective on their inner processes and patterns. Writing about their breathwork journey allows individuals to capture insights, revelations, and shifts in consciousness that may arise during the practice. Journaling also provides a tangible record of progress and growth over time, allowing individuals to track their journey of self-discovery.

2. Body Sensations and Emotional Release:

Breathwork often involves becoming attuned to subtle body sensations and emotional cues that arise during the practice. By tuning into these sensations and allowing them to be fully felt and expressed, individuals can facilitate emotional release, healing, and integration. Through breathwork, individuals can access deeper layers of emotion stored in the body, allowing them to release tension, trauma, and stuck energy. As individuals become more adept at recognizing and processing their emotions through breathwork, they develop greater emotional resilience and well-being.

3. Guided Imagery and Visualization:

Incorporating guided imagery and visualization into breathwork sessions enhances self-reflection and inner exploration. Guided imagery allows individuals to embark on vivid sensory experiences and symbolic journeys, tapping into their subconscious mind and accessing deeper layers of insight and creativity. By guiding individuals through visualizations that resonate with their personal goals and intentions, facilitators can help individuals gain clarity, inspiration, and direction in their lives. Visualizations may focus on areas such as self-compassion, inner strength, or visioning the future, empowering individuals to manifest their deepest desires and aspirations.

4. Integration and Application:

The insights gained through breathwork can be integrated into daily life through intentional reflection and application. Individuals can reflect on their breathwork experiences, identifying key insights, themes, and patterns that emerge. They can then apply these insights to their daily routines, relationships, and decision-making processes. By integrating breathwork into their self-care practices, individuals cultivate greater self-awareness, resilience, and well-being, leading to a more fulfilling and purposeful life.

In summary, using breathwork for self-reflection provides individuals with a powerful tool for exploring their inner world, gaining insight into their thoughts and emotions, and fostering personal growth and transformation. Whether through journaling, body awareness, guided imagery, or integration practices, breathwork offers a pathway to greater self-awareness, authenticity, and well-being.

CHAPTER 16: Cultivating a Breath Practice

In this chapter, we explore the process of cultivating a breath practice, focusing on how individuals can develop a consistent routine and overcome challenges in establishing and maintaining their breathwork practice.

Developing a Consistent Breath Routine

Establishing a consistent breath routine is fundamental to harnessing the full benefits of breathwork. Consistency not only allows individuals to deepen their practice but also ensures that they integrate breathwork seamlessly into their daily lives. Here's how to develop a consistent breath routine:

- **Set Clear Intentions:**

Start by defining your objectives for incorporating breathwork into your routine. Ask yourself why you want to practice breathwork and what specific outcomes you hope to achieve. Whether it's reducing stress, improving focus, or enhancing overall well-being, clarifying your intentions provides a guiding light for your practice.

- **Create a Dedicated Space:**

Designate a tranquil and comfortable space for your breathwork practice. This area should be free from distractions and conducive to relaxation. Whether it's a corner of your home, a cushion in your living room, or a peaceful outdoor spot, having a designated space helps signal to your mind that it's time for practice, fostering consistency and focus.

- **Establish a Routine:**

Consistency is key to developing a sustainable breath practice. Schedule regular times for your practice, whether it's daily, several times a week, or weekly. Choose times that align with your schedule and energy levels, making it easier to stick to your routine. Treat your breathwork sessions as non-negotiable appointments with yourself, prioritizing them like any other important commitment.

- **Start Small:**

Begin with short practice sessions to make it easier to integrate breathwork into your routine. Even just a few minutes of focused breathing can yield significant benefits. Starting small allows you to build momentum gradually and prevents overwhelm. As you become more comfortable with your practice, you can gradually increase the duration and intensity of your sessions.

- **Find What Works for You:**

Explore different breathwork techniques and styles to find what resonates with you. There are various approaches to breathwork, including mindfulness breathing, pranayama, and guided breathwork. Experiment with different techniques to discover what feels most natural and effective for you. Tailor your practice to suit your preferences, needs, and goals, ensuring that it aligns with your unique lifestyle and personality.

- **Stay Flexible and Adaptive:**

While consistency is essential, it's also important to remain flexible and adaptive in your approach to breathwork. Life can be unpredictable, and there may be times when your schedule or circumstances prevent you from sticking to your usual routine. Instead of becoming discouraged, be willing to adapt your practice to accommodate changing circumstances. This might involve practicing at different times of the day or adjusting the duration of your sessions as needed.

- **Track Your Progress:**

Keep track of your breathwork practice to monitor your progress and stay motivated. Consider maintaining a journal where you can record details about your practice, such as the techniques used, the duration of each session, and any insights or experiences that arise. Tracking your progress allows you to celebrate your successes, identify areas for growth, and stay committed to your practice over the long term.

By following these steps and incorporating breathwork into your daily routine, you can cultivate a consistent and rewarding practice that supports your overall well-being and personal growth journey. Remember that consistency is key, and even small steps taken consistently can lead to significant transformation over time.

Overcoming Challenges in Establishing a Breath Practice

Establishing a breath practice can be immensely rewarding, but it's not without its challenges. However, with patience, perseverance, and the right strategies, individuals can overcome these obstacles and build a sustainable breath practice that supports their well-being. Here's how to navigate common challenges in establishing a breath practice:

- **Lack of Time:**

One of the most common challenges individuals face is finding time for breathwork amidst busy schedules.

To overcome this challenge:

- **Prioritize Your Practice:** Treat your breathwork practice as a non-negotiable part of your self-care routine. Schedule it into your day just like you would any other important commitment.

- **Start Small:** Begin with short, manageable sessions, even if it's just a few minutes each day. Gradually increase the duration as you become more comfortable with your practice.

- **Resistance or Distractions:**

Resistance or distractions during breathwork can hinder progress and consistency.

To address this challenge:

- **Acknowledge and Accept:** Notice any resistance or distractions that arise during your practice without judgment. Accept them as natural parts of the process and gently guide your focus back to your breath.

- **Set Clear Boundaries:** Minimize distractions by creating a dedicated space for your practice and setting clear boundaries with yourself and others during this time.

- **Inconsistency:**

Maintaining consistency in your breath practice can be challenging, especially when life gets busy or unpredictable.

To foster greater consistency:

- **Revisit Your Intentions:** Reflect on your reasons for practicing breathwork and the benefits you've experienced so far. Use these insights as motivation to recommit to your practice.

- **Find Accountability Partners:** Share your breathwork goals with friends, family, or a supportive community. Having accountability partners can help keep you motivated and on track with your practice.

- **Perfectionism:**

Striving for perfection in your breath practice can create unnecessary pressure and hinder progress.

To overcome perfectionism:

- **Embrace Imperfection**: Remember that breathwork is a journey, not a destination. Embrace the process of learning and growth, and allow yourself to make mistakes along the way.

- **Cultivate Self-Compassion:** Practice self-compassion and kindness towards yourself, especially when facing challenges or setbacks. Treat yourself with the same understanding and empathy you would offer to a close friend.

- **Lack of Guidance:**

Without proper guidance, individuals may struggle to know where to start or how to progress in their breath practice.

To address this challenge:

- **Seek Resources:** Explore books, online courses, workshops, or guided meditation apps that offer instruction and guidance on breathwork techniques.

- **Find a Mentor or Teacher:** Consider working with a breathwork teacher or mentor who can provide personalized guidance, support, and encouragement on your breathwork journey.

By implementing these strategies and approaches, individuals can overcome the challenges of establishing a breath practice and cultivate a sustainable routine that supports their overall well-being and personal growth. Remember that consistency, patience, and self-compassion are key to navigating the ups and downs of the breathwork journey.

CHAPTER 17: Breath and Connection to Nature

In this chapter, we explore the profound connection between breath and nature, and how immersing oneself in natural environments can enhance breath awareness and deepen one's breathwork practice.

Nature Walks and Breath Awareness

Nature walks provide a beautiful opportunity to immerse oneself in the natural world and deepen breath awareness. Here's how nature walks can be conducive to cultivating mindful breath awareness:

1. Mindful Observation:

During a nature walk, individuals can focus on their breath while observing the sights, sounds, and sensations of the environment around them. With each step, they can tune into the rhythm of their breath, noticing how it synchronizes with their movement and the natural world.

By cultivating mindfulness, individuals develop a deeper connection to their breath and the present moment.

2. Deep Breathing:

Nature walks offer a serene setting for practicing deep breathing exercises. Participants can pause along the trail to take deep, intentional breaths, inhaling fresh air deeply into their lungs and exhaling slowly to release tension and stress. Deep breathing in nature can promote relaxation, rejuvenation, and a sense of inner peace.

3. Engagement of the Senses:

Nature walks engage all the senses, providing ample opportunities to connect with the breath on a sensory level. Participants can inhale the earthy scent of the forest, listen to the soothing sounds of flowing water or birdsong, feel the gentle breeze against their skin, and observe the vibrant colors and textures of the landscape. By fully engaging the senses, individuals deepen their awareness of their breath and its connection to the natural world.

4. Gratitude Practice:

Nature walks offer a chance to express gratitude for the beauty and abundance of the natural world. Participants can cultivate a sense of awe and appreciation with each breath, acknowledging the interconnectedness of all living beings and the gifts that nature provides. Gratitude practice during nature walks fosters a deeper connection to the breath and instills a sense of reverence for the earth and its ecosystems.

Overall, nature walks serve as a powerful backdrop for cultivating breath awareness and mindfulness. By tuning into the rhythm of their breath amidst the beauty of the outdoors, individuals deepen their connection to themselves, each other, and the natural world, fostering a sense of peace, balance, and harmony.

Breath Practices in Natural Settings

Practicing breathwork in natural settings can deepen one's connection to the environment and enhance the benefits of breathwork techniques. Here are some ways to incorporate breath practices into natural settings:

1. Pranayama in the Outdoors:

Pranayama, or yogic breathing techniques, can be particularly impactful when practiced outdoors. Find a quiet and peaceful spot in nature, such as a forest clearing or a tranquil meadow, to practice pranayama. Techniques like alternate nostril breathing, ujjayi breath, or kapalabhati can be performed amidst the sights, sounds, and scents of the natural world. Practicing pranayama outdoors allows individuals to synchronize their breath with the rhythms of nature, promoting a sense of harmony and balance.

2. Grounding Breathwork:

Grounding breathwork exercises are especially effective when practiced in direct contact with the earth. Find a patch of soft grass, a sandy beach, or a moss-covered rock to sit or lie down on. Close your eyes and visualize your breath flowing down into the earth with each inhale, grounding you deeply into the earth's energy. As you exhale, release any tension or worries, allowing them to be absorbed by the earth beneath you. Grounding breathwork in natural settings helps individuals feel supported, stable, and connected to the earth's nurturing energy.

3. Breath Meditation:

Nature provides an ideal backdrop for breath-focused meditation. Find a secluded spot with natural beauty, such as a serene lakeside or a peaceful grove of trees, to practice breath meditation. Close your eyes and bring your attention to the sensation of your breath as it moves in and out of your body. Notice how the sights, sounds, and sensations of nature gently guide your breath, deepening your sense of connection to the present moment. Breath meditation in natural settings fosters a profound sense of peace, tranquility, and presence.

4. Breath Rituals:

Create simple breath rituals that honor the natural world and deepen your connection to it. Gather natural objects such as leaves, stones, or flowers to use as focal points for your breathwork practice. Find a quiet spot in nature to sit or stand, holding your chosen objects in your hands. With each breath, infuse your intentions of harmony, balance, and connection into the objects, allowing them to absorb the energy of the earth and the elements. Breath rituals in natural settings offer a sacred space for reflection, intention-setting, and communion with the natural world.

Incorporating breath practices into natural settings amplifies the benefits of breathwork, fostering a deeper sense of connection, presence, and vitality. Whether practicing pranayama, grounding breathwork, breath meditation, or breath rituals, individuals can harness the healing power of nature to support their breathwork journey and enhance their overall well-being.

CHAPTER 18: Teaching Breath to Others

In this chapter, we explore the art of sharing breath techniques with others and leading breathwork workshops to empower individuals to cultivate greater well-being and self-awareness through breath.

Sharing Breath Techniques with Others

Teaching breath techniques to others is a meaningful way to empower individuals to enhance their well-being and cultivate mindfulness in their lives. Here are some effective strategies for sharing breath techniques with others:

1. Demonstrate and Explain:

Start by demonstrating the breath techniques you wish to teach, providing clear and concise instructions for each step. Use simple language and visual aids, such as diagrams or illustrations, to help participants understand the mechanics of each breath technique. Break down the technique into manageable components, and demonstrate each step slowly and methodically.

2. Provide Guidance and Support:

Offer guidance and support as participants practice the breath techniques. Encourage them to explore different variations and modifications to find what works best for their unique needs and preferences. Be attentive to their questions, concerns, and experiences, providing reassurance and encouragement along the way. Offer adjustments or modifications as needed to ensure that participants feel comfortable and supported in their practice.

3. Encourage Exploration and Experimentation:

Encourage participants to explore and experiment with the breath techniques outside of the teaching session. Offer suggestions for integrating breathwork into their daily routines and provide resources for further learning and exploration, such as recommended readings, online resources, or guided meditation apps. Encourage participants to keep an open mind and approach their breath practice with curiosity and self-compassion.

4. Create a Safe and Supportive Environment:

Foster a safe and supportive environment where participants feel comfortable sharing their experiences and asking questions. Create a sense of community and connection among participants by fostering open communication and mutual respect. Encourage peer support and collaboration, and create opportunities for participants to share their insights, challenges, and successes with one another. Emphasize the importance of confidentiality and respect for each individual's journey.

5. Provide Follow-Up Resources:

Offer follow-up resources and support to participants after the teaching session ends. Provide handouts or digital resources summarizing the breath techniques taught during the session, along with additional tips and suggestions for incorporating breathwork into daily life. Offer access to recordings of guided breathwork sessions or online communities where participants can connect with fellow practitioners and continue their breathwork journey.

By effectively sharing breath techniques with others, individuals can empower them to harness the transformative power of breath and cultivate greater mindfulness, resilience, and well-being in their lives. Through clear instruction, guidance, and support, participants can develop the skills and confidence to incorporate breathwork into their daily routines and experience the myriad benefits it offers.

Leading Breathwork Workshops

Leading breathwork workshops is a powerful way to create a supportive environment for individuals to explore breath techniques, deepen their practice, and cultivate greater well-being. Here are some effective strategies for leading breathwork workshops:

1. Design a Structured Curriculum:

Start by developing a structured curriculum that covers a variety of breath techniques, ranging from basic mindfulness breathing to more advanced pranayama practices. Consider the needs, interests, and experience levels of your participants when designing the curriculum, and ensure that it provides a balanced and comprehensive overview of breathwork practices.

2. Facilitate Experiential Learning:

Prioritize experiential learning by providing ample opportunities for participants to practice the breath techniques firsthand. Incorporate guided exercises, meditations, and group activities to deepen participants' understanding and embodiment of the breathwork practices. Encourage participants to actively engage with the material and share their insights and experiences with the group.

3. Offer Individualized Support:

Recognize that each participant may have unique experiences, challenges, and preferences when it comes to breathwork. Offer individualized support and guidance, tailoring your approach to meet the needs of each participant. Be responsive to feedback and adjust your teaching style accordingly. Create a safe and non-judgmental space where participants feel comfortable sharing their experiences and asking questions.

4. Cultivate a Transformative Experience:

Set an intention for the workshop and hold space for deep exploration and self-discovery. Create an immersive and transformative experience for participants by incorporating elements of ritual, ceremony, or mindfulness into the workshop format. Foster a sense of trust and vulnerability among participants, allowing them to open up to the healing potential of breathwork. Encourage participants to approach the workshop with an open mind and heart, and to embrace whatever arises during the practice.

5. Follow Up and Continued Support:

Offer follow-up resources and support to participants after the workshop ends. Provide access to recordings, reading materials, or online communities where participants can continue their breathwork journey and stay connected with fellow practitioners. Follow up with participants individually to check in on their progress and offer additional support or guidance as needed. Create opportunities for ongoing learning and growth, such as advanced workshops or retreats, to support participants in deepening their practice over time.

By effectively leading breathwork workshops, individuals can create a supportive and transformative environment where participants can explore the power of breath and cultivate greater mindfulness, resilience, and well-being. Through structured curriculum, experiential learning, individualized support, and ongoing follow-up, workshops can serve as catalysts for profound personal growth and transformation.

Conclusion

In conclusion, breathwork offers a profound pathway to enhanced well-being, inner peace, and self-awareness. Throughout this journey, we have explored key concepts and practices that underscore the transformative power of breath. Let us recap some of these essential insights:

1. Understanding the Significance of Breath: Breath is not merely a physiological function but a gateway to deeper connection with ourselves and the world around us. By becoming aware of our breath, we tap into its potential to calm the mind, regulate emotions, and cultivate presence.

2. Exploring Breath Techniques: From conscious breathing and pranayama to guided meditation and breath-centric movement, a diverse array of breath techniques empowers us to explore the many dimensions of our breath. Each technique offers unique benefits and insights into our inner landscape.

3. Recognizing the Connection Between Breath and Well-being: Stress, emotions, and physical health are intricately linked to our breath patterns. By harnessing the power of breath, we can mitigate stress, enhance emotional resilience, and improve respiratory function, thus nurturing holistic well-being.

4. Sharing the Gift of Breath: As we deepen our own breath practice, let us share this transformative gift with others. Whether through teaching breath techniques or leading workshops, we have the opportunity to inspire and support individuals on their journey toward greater vitality and self-discovery.

As we conclude this exploration of breath, I encourage each of you to continue your journey of exploration and practice. Embrace breath as a lifelong companion and guide, leading you toward greater presence, clarity, and joy. May your breath be a source of inspiration, resilience, and connection as you navigate the beauty and complexity of life.

Inhale deeply, exhale fully, and embrace the transformative power of your breath. The journey continues, one breath at a time.